THE AMERICAN DIABETES ASSOCIATION
vegetarian cookbook

SATISFYING, BOLD, AND FLAVORFUL RECIPES FROM THE GARDEN

By CHEF STEVEN PETUSEVSKY
Author of *The Whole Foods Market Cookbook*

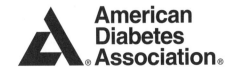

American
Diabetes
Association®

Director, Book Publishing, Abe Ogden; *Managing Editor*, Greg Guthrie; *Acquisitions Editor*, Victor Van Beuren; *Editor*, Rebekah Renshaw; *Production Manager*, Melissa Sprott; *Composition and Cover Design*, Jenn French Designs, LLC.; *Photographer*, Renee Comet; *Printer*, Marquis Imprimeur.

Printed in Canada
1 3 5 7 9 10 8 6 4 2

The suggestions and information contained in this publication are generally consistent with the *Clinical Practice Recommendations* and other policies of the American Diabetes Association, but they do not represent the policy or position of the Association or any of its boards or committees. Reasonable steps have been taken to ensure the accuracy of the information presented. However, the American Diabetes Association cannot ensure the safety or efficacy of any product or service described in this publication. Individuals are advised to consult a physician or other appropriate health care professional before undertaking any diet or exercise program or taking any medication referred to in this publication. Professionals must use and apply their own professional judgment, experience, and training and should not rely solely on the information contained in this publication before prescribing any diet, exercise, or medication. The American Diabetes Association—its officers, directors, employees, volunteers, and members—assumes no responsibility or liability for personal orother injury, loss, or damage that may result from the suggestions or information in this publication.

⊗ The paper in this publication meets the requirements of the ANSI Standard Z39.48-1992 (permanence of paper).

ADA titles may be purchased for business or promotional use or for special sales. To purchase more than 50 copies of this book at a discount, or for custom editions of this book with your logo, contact the American Diabetes Association at the address below, at booksales@diabetes.org, or by calling 703-299-2046.

American Diabetes Association
1701 North Beauregard Street
Alexandria, Virginia 22311

DOI: 10.2337/97815804048777

Library of Congress Cataloging-in-Publication Data
Petusevsky, Steve.
The American Diabetes Association vegetarian cookbook / Steven Petusevsky.
pages cm
Includes bibliographical references and index.
ISBN 978-1-58040-487-7 (alk. paper)
1. Diabetes--Diet therapy--Recipes. 2. Vegetarian cooking. 3. Cooking (Vegetables) I. American Diabetes Association. II. Title.
RC662.P47 2013
641.5'6314--dc23

2013008330

table of contents

acknowledgments

Book acknowledgments are always difficult because it means that the book, a true labor of love, is finished. There are also so many people to thank and I'm always afraid I will miss someone important who either put up with me over the last year, or in some way helped the outcome of this book.

With that said, I want to thank Abe Ogden, Rebekah Renshaw, and Greg Guthrie at the American Diabetes Association for presenting me with the opportunity to write this book and allowing me to reach so many people who will benefit from these pages. Thanks to Renee Comet of Renee Comet Photography and food stylist Lisa Cherkasky for their brilliant photographs. My hope is to positively affect many readers and perhaps inspire them to begin new traditions with their families and friends. I want them to know creative healthful food is simple, beautiful, and delicious.

I also want to thank Lori, my better half (and a vegetarian), for always being supportive and encouraging me to eat my vegetables, for willingly consuming everything I cook, and for being honest when it came time for feedback.

My agent and friend for many years, Beth Shepard, made this book possible, and I cherish her as a life ally. Terry Dalton introduced me to a new and enlightened way of cooking nearly 25 years ago at the Unicorn Village in North Miami and, fortunately, he was 30 years ahead of his time. Sara Baer Sinnott and the Oldways Foundation led me around the world and opened up the notion of true global cuisine. Over the years, they have inspired me to earnestly seek authentic roots cooking globally. In parts of the world I never dreamed I would actually be, let alone cook, I learned that great vegetarian food should be "great food", not labeled just vegetarian. I wanted to thank my old friends Bobby and Rachel Koeningsberg for letting me camp out for weeks at a time in their beautiful cottage in Colorado while I cooked many of these recipes. I will never forget some of these "farm to table" dinners. Enjoy cooking these recipes as much as I have enjoyed creating them for you.

Chef Steve

introduction

Why another cookbook, and a vegetarian cookbook at that? Even when you take into consideration the fact that vegetarian cooking—really great vegetarian cooking—can be intimidating for many home cooks, I wanted to offer more than just recipes. The essence and message of this book is personal. Two years ago, I was diagnosed with "prediabetes"—blood glucose levels that are higher than normal but not yet high enough to be diagnosed as diabetes. I also had high blood pressure and high cholesterol. I tried to justify this prognosis to myself, shrugging off any personal responsibility. After all, I've been a professional chef my whole life. I literally fell apart. I had been living in the Midwest, working on a three-year contract, away from family, friends, and everything dear to me. My solution and consolation became making poor food choices. Along with the cheese, fried cheese curds, deep fried fish, and donuts, I lived in the epicenter of beer production. Clearly that didn't help the situation.

I moved back to my home state of Florida after my contract was up, knowing that something was terribly wrong with my internal chemistry. My doctor immediately put me on several medications and routine blood work to monitor my progress. I found the whole situation embarrassing, invasive, and depressing. How could this happen to me, the guy who had spent the last several decades touting healthy cuisine? The truth is that what happened to me happens every day—it may have happened to you, your partner, a friend, or your kids.

Flash forward two years later and I can honestly tell you that I have never felt better. After losing more than 30 pounds, I'm off most of the medications, and although I have more work to do, I am now walking the walk and following my own advice. I am not a total vegetarian; however, I eat vegetarian meals at least four days a week. I exercise regularly and can tell you that my attitude has completely changed for the better. My life has improved greatly and I'm managing my prediabetes with many of the recipes you'll find in this book. If a chef who lives, eats, and breathes food 24/7 can make such dramatic changes in his life, you can too.

No one wants to sacrifice flavor for health. This is the best thing about the recipes in this book. They are easy to make, have incredible flavor, and will never bore you or your friends and family. These recipes rely on simple, fresh, and seasonal ingredients and how they relate to each other through taste, texture, color, and flavor harmony. Chefs know this as the Asian 5-Flavor Principle, which universally guides our taste buds. Sweet, sour, salty, spicy, and bitter are the primal elements of taste that, when carefully balanced, resonate together to make us simply say WOW with every forkful.

For me, it's flavor first! Many cultures worldwide are essentially vegetarian-friendly although they do not label or categorize their cuisine as vegetarian. It's just a part of their culture.

There are several classifications of vegetarians. The most common definition describes any diet that favors plant-based foods and discourages eating any animal ingredients. Many vegetarians maintain a restrictive regimen excluding all animal flesh and animal byproducts, such as dairy and eggs.

Vegans do not even consume animal products like honey. Some less restrictive vegetarian diets, such as lacto-ovo vegetarians, permit eggs and most dairy products.

Some classifications of "-tarians"—often self-styled—are a bit looser. Flexitarians regularly seek vegetarian foods, but also eat meat. Pescetarians often call themselves vegetarians, but eat fish—just not meat or poultry.

Fruitarians are a subgroup of vegans who thrive on the fruit of trees, shrubs, etc., a diet that may or may not also include nuts, seeds, pulses, and root vegetables.

Vegetarians must consume a variety of plant-based foods, including grains, nuts, seeds, fruits, vegetables, legumes, and oils, with the greatest challenge being consuming enough protein and certain valuable vitamins and minerals.

For many of these diets, a minimum amount of processed foods—if any—is a given.

With that said, my advice to you is to enjoy these recipes, allow yourself to connect to the seasons and ethnic influences of the recipes, and above all, openly and proudly share the finished results with family and friends. Perhaps you'll start new dinner table traditions and rekindle your own relationship with healthful, flavorful, and wonderful vegetarian meals.

To your health!
Chef Steve

vegetarian pantry 101

Creating a vegetarian pantry is a process—an evolution of sorts and collection of favorite herbs and spices, condiments, dried pastas, legumes, canned goods, and more. My personal pantry has evolved over the years and I find that I constantly add new items that intrigue and inspire my cooking. A vegetarian pantry is alive and grows with experience as you create recipes that become favorites and regularly make their way onto your family dinner table. These suggestions will help you build the foundation of your pantry.

There was a time when stocking a vegetarian pantry was challenging. You had to go to a dozen little stores to find what you needed, and even then, many items were spotty. Luckily, all this has changed. You can find everything you need in almost every large supermarket or natural foods grocer. Ethnic markets have also sprung up around the country offering ingredients from every culture of the globe. Condiments, sauces, spices, pastas, and even fresh produce from around the world can be found in many neighborhood ethnic stores allow us to cook once obscure global recipes in our home kitchens. With the rising popularity of vegetarian cooking, whole grains and alternative proteins are also a breeze to find. Here's my pick for a perfect pantry offering—these are all items that you would typically find in my pantry.

PASTA
I separate pasta into two major categories: semolina, the traditional flour for pasta making; and whole grains, which include all the other grains, such as rice, quinoa, spelt, kamut, and buckwheat flour pasta. You will want to experiment with all of them.

BEANS AND LEGUMES
There are wonderful selections of beans and legumes available canned, jarred, and dried. I seem to use the canned versions most often as they are convenient. Make sure that you rinse canned beans or legumes with cold water to remove the sodium that they are packed in. Go ahead and experiment with cooking your own dried beans or legumes from scratch— it's time consuming but often worth it for their fresh rich taste.

Garbanzo or chickpeas, cannellini beans, black beans, adzuki, and kidney beans are my go to beans. There are also heirloom and unusual beans such as Appaloosa, Anasazi, and dozens of others to try. These are only available dried. Each has a different character and flavor to offer.

Green lentils and orange lentils are always fun for salads and soups as well. They are simple to cook from a dried state.

CONDIMENTS

Seasoning blends can be found in every market now, which combine various herbs and spices. Just start collecting them to find ones that you like. Curry, Italian, Mexican, and Asian blends are some common ones. Lemon pepper and other salt-free blends abound. Be adventurous and try them.

Some other "must haves" include:

> Sriracha, a spicy Asian catsup is my favorite and a must have
> Sambal, a spicy chili paste
> Tamari or soy sauce
> Ponzu, a citrus soy sauce
> Hoisin sauce
> Dijon and stone-ground mustard
> Harissa, a Moroccan spice paste
> Sesame seeds, both black and white
> Smoked paprika, either spicy or sweet

VINEGARS AND OILS

> Canola oil
> Grapeseed oil
> Extra virgin olive oil
> Dark roasted sesame oil
> Specialty oils for special meals: truffle oil, hazelnut oil, walnut oil, spicy chili oil
> Cider vinegar
> Red wine vinegar
> Balsamic vinegar
> Rice vinegar

ON FLAVORED VINEGARS AND OILS

They are both simple to make. Use 2 cups of olive or canola oil; put a handful of your favorite spices such as peppercorns, garlic cloves, hot chili flakes, fresh herb stalks, bay leaves, etc., into the oil. Bring to a slight boil and turn off the heat. Allow the oil to sit overnight and then pour it into a bottle, adding some of the flavorings.

Use the same procedure to create flavored oils. My favorite is Asian spiced oil, which I use for all my Asian-inspired dishes; 2 cups canola or grapeseed oil, 1 cup dark roasted sesame oil, some hot chili flakes or whole dried chilis, 3 slices of fresh ginger, 3 garlic cloves, a few star anise buds or a cinnamon stick.

GRAINS

All grains have their own flavor, character, cooking time, and ratio of liquid to grains when they are cooked. Follow instructions for each and you will end up with some great new favorites. Although there are many more varieties, here are my go-to grains:

- Quinoa
- Kamut
- Faro
- Spelt
- Amaranth
- Bulgur wheat
- Wheat berries
- Barley
- Oats

ETHNIC

This is your chance to go wild and be playful. Visit local ethnic markets and after reading the labels, try a few items at a time until you build your own personal favorites. The reason I suggest reading the labels is sometimes there are hidden ingredients you don't want, like sugar, MSG, and high levels of sodium. I frequent Asian, Indian, Latin, and Mediterranean markets for ingredient inspiration. Along with spices and condiments ethnic markets offer a really unusual selection of pasta varieties, breads, soup mixes, and fresh hard-to-find produce.

ALTERNATIVE PROTEINS

Where once tofu and tempeh were the only major sources of vegetarian protein, the offerings have expanded with the demand. Here are my favorites:

- Flavored or smoked tofu, ones with sprouted grains, or even in sauce ready to eat.
- Spiced or marinated tempeh, which comes in a variety of flavors.
- Wheat gluten-based proteins such as seitan, or branded wheat, and soy gluten items such as gardein, one of my favorites.
- Soy-based "ground beef," vegetarian protein crumbles, sausage, chorizo, and cutlets. I think most of these products are great to cook with and really expand the vegetarian dinner choices.

CHAPTER 1
Soups: Both Warmed and Chilled

Soups are liquid pleasure. They are forgiving and almost any recipe can be altered to use up little bits and pieces of vegetables, leftover beans or grains, or maybe even that pile of overripe tomatoes from summer's garden harvest. Soups are comforting and wholesome and, depending on the season, soups make a complete meal when served with a loaf of warm bread or a tossed green salad. Gone are the days when soups were thickened with lots of flour and fat; the soups you'll find here are rich in flavor and texture from vegetables and grains and wonderfully fragrant herbs and spices. The fact that these soups are vegetarian is just a bonus to your good health.

Soup encourages us to prepare and taste the authentic flavors of other lands. Whether it is the spicy aroma of chili peppers and cracked cumin, or the sweet smell of ginger, star anise, and lemongrass wafting through our home, soup is powerful food.

A pot of simmering soup can evoke emotion and stir memories of the past. There is perhaps no greater antidote when we feel run down. On the other hand, well-made chilled soup refreshes the soul and brings us back to life when we are overheated. A chilled bowl of gazpacho revitalizes our spirit while a steaming bowl of Miso noodle soup literally cures our ills.

As you cook your way through this chapter, enjoy these favorite recipes and hopefully some of them will become your family traditions for years to come.

energizing minestrone

 10 servings

 2 cups

Full of nutrient-rich vegetables and fiber-rich beans, this minestrone will keep you energized all day. You can use any type of canned beans and small pasta shapes in this recipe. Often fresh or canned chopped tomatoes are added, but they are not a requirement.

1 tablespoon olive oil

1 cup chopped onions

1 cup chopped celery

1 cup chopped carrots

3 cloves minced garlic

1 tablespoon dried oregano

2 cups peeled, seeded, and chopped calabasa or butternut squash

2 cups peeled (1/2-inch cubes) Yukon gold potatoes

2 quarts low-sodium vegetable broth or water

3 cups chopped kale, cabbage, or spinach

1 (16-ounce) can cannellini beans or chickpeas, drained well and rinsed

1 cup cooked whole-wheat pasta (such as orzo, small shells, ditalini, or elbows)

Salt, to taste

Fresh-ground black pepper, to taste

1/2 cup chopped fresh basil

1/2 cup shredded Parmesan cheese

1 Heat oil in a large saucepan over medium-high heat. Add the onions, celery, carrots, garlic, and oregano. Sauté 3 minutes until vegetables are soft.

2 Add the squash and potatoes and continue to sauté 1 minute. Add the broth or water and bring to a boil. Reduce heat and simmer 15 minutes.

3 Add the kale, beans, and cooked pasta. Simmer another 10 minutes. Season with salt and pepper. Add basil and serve garnished with Parmesan cheese.

 CHEF STEVE'S TIP:

Always add fresh herbs last to preserve aroma and flavor.

EXCHANGES/CHOICES 1 Starch | 2 Vegetable | 1/2 Fat

Calories 140 | Calories from Fat 20 | Total Fat 2.5 g | Saturated Fat 0.6 g | Trans Fat 0.0 g
Cholesterol 0 mg | Sodium 200 mg | Potassium 565 mg | Total Carbohydrate 25 g
Dietary Fiber 5 g | Sugars 6 g | Protein 6 g | Phosphorus 170 mg

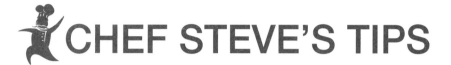

CHEF STEVE'S TIPS

beans

Beans are an important ingredient in vegetarian cooking. They contain more protein than any other food in the vegetable kingdom—1/2 cup cooked dried beans equals the amount of protein found in 1 ounce of lean meat. Bean protein is unlike the complete protein found in seafood, poultry, and beef as it lacks some of the vital amino acids. When grains, seeds, or dairy are eaten in combination with beans, a high-quality complete protein source is formed. Beans are also one of the best sources of soluble fiber, which may lower levels of serum cholesterol.

Canned and jarred beans are a good alternative to dried and are less time-consuming to prepare. To reduce the sodium content in canned beans, make sure you rinse the beans well in a colander before using.

holiday yucca stew with black beans, cilantro, and lime

 8 servings

 1 1/2 cups

Yucca is soul satisfying. When combined with spicy jalapeño, tart tomato, lime, and cilantro, this hearty root vegetable absorbs the taste of these ingredients and lightly thickens the soup naturally.

1 (12-ounce) package frozen yucca

6 quarts water or low-sodium vegetable stock

2 tablespoons olive oil

2 cloves garlic, minced

1 small red onion, chopped

1 jalapeño pepper, seeded and minced

1 large tomato, chopped

1 cup low-sodium tomato juice

1 (15-ounce) can black beans, rinsed and drained

2 tablespoons lime juice

1/4 cup minced cilantro

1/4 cup shelled pumpkin seeds

1 small avocado, peeled, pitted, and diced

1 Place yucca in a 2-quart saucepan and cover with water or stock. Bring to a boil, reduce heat, and simmer 12–15 minutes until tender. Drain and let cool. Cut into bite-sized pieces and set aside.

2 Heat oil in a large nonreactive skillet or sauté pan over medium heat. Add garlic, onions, and jalapeños, and sauté 5 minutes until tender.

3 Add tomatoes, tomato juice, beans, and yucca. Bring to a boil, reduce heat, and simmer 10 minutes. Add lime juice and cilantro. Serve in large bowls garnished with pumpkin seeds and diced avocado.

EXCHANGES/CHOICES 1 1/2 Starch | 1 Vegetable | 1 1/2 Fat

Calories 200 | Calories from Fat 65 | Total Fat 7.0 g | Saturated Fat 1.1 g | Trans Fat 0.0 g
Cholesterol 0 mg | Sodium 50 mg | Potassium 470 mg | Total Carbohydrate 30 g
Dietary Fiber 5 g | Sugars 4 g | Protein 5 g | Phosphorus 120 mg

pumpkin chowder with toasted pepitas

 8 servings

 1 cup

This chowder is rich and full of bold tropical flavor. You can leave it chunky as I do, or purée it if you like it smooth and creamy. Sometimes I substitute 1 cup of the vegetable broth or water for a cup of light coconut milk for a bit of extra richness.

2 pounds calabaza squash, peeled and chopped

8 cups water or low-sodium vegetable broth

1 large tomato, chopped

1 medium onion, chopped

1 medium green bell pepper, chopped

1 jalapeño pepper or scotch bonnet chili, seeded and minced

1 tablespoon minced gingerroot

8 scallions, chopped

3 sprigs fresh thyme or 1 teaspoon dried

1/4 cup chopped cilantro

Juice of 1 lime

Salt, to taste

Toasted Pepitas (see box)

1 Place squash, broth, tomatoes, onion, pepper, ginger root, scallions, and thyme sprigs or dried thyme in a nonreactive large saucepan. Bring to a boil, reduce heat, and simmer uncovered for 45 minutes, stirring occasionally, until all ingredients are tender.

2 Add cilantro, lime juice, and salt. Remove thyme stems before serving. Garnish each bowl of soup with pepitas (see box) before serving. Makes about 2 quarts.

EXCHANGES/CHOICES (without pepitas) 1/2 Starch | 1 Vegetable

Calories 50 | Calories from Fat 0 | Total Fat 0.0 g | Saturated Fat 0.1 g | Trans Fat 0.0 g
Cholesterol 0 mg | Sodium 20 mg | Potassium 335 mg | Total Carbohydrate 12 g
Dietary Fiber 4 g | Sugars 5 g | Protein 2 g | Phosphorus 50 mg

TOASTED PEPITAS

 8 servings

 1 ounce

2 teaspoons canola oil

1 cup shelled pumpkin seeds

Salt, to taste

Serve as a healthy table snack. Dust them with a bit of Cajun seasoning for a bit of heat.

1 In a nonstick sauté pan or skillet, heat oil over medium heat. Add pumpkin seeds and sauté 3 minutes until they begin to brown and "pop." Sprinkle with salt and use as a soup garnish or eat out of hand.

EXCHANGES/CHOICES 2 Fat

Calories 95 | Calories from Fat 70 | Total Fat 8.0 g
Saturated Fat 1.3 g | Trans Fat 0.0 g | Cholesterol 0 mg
Sodium 0 mg | Potassium 115 mg | Total Carbohydrate 2 g
Dietary Fiber 1 g | Sugars 0 g | Protein 4 g | Phosphorus 175 mg

greek egg and lemon soup

 8 servings

 1/8 recipe

I was first introduced to this soup on the island of Chios. It's a staple throughout Greece with a warm and sunny flavor much like the people who live there.

8 cups low-sodium vegetable broth

1 cup white basmati rice or orzo

2 whole garlic cloves, peeled

5 egg yolks

Zest of 1 lemon

Juice of 3 lemons

Freshly ground black pepper, to taste

1 Combine the vegetable broth with rice or orzo and whole garlic cloves. Bring to a boil, reduce heat, and simmer uncovered for 20 minutes, or until tender. Discard garlic cloves.

2 In a large mixing bowl, combine yolks, lemon zest, lemon juice, and ground pepper. Whisk until well combined.

3 When the orzo or rice is tender, ladle about 2 cups hot broth into a large mixing bowl. While you whisk the egg mixture, very slowly drizzle the 2 cups hot broth into the egg yolk mixture; if you add it too quickly you will scramble the egg yolks. This is what you want to avoid. Continue whisking and adding liquid to the egg yolks until the mixing bowl is empty.

4 Remove the saucepan with the orzo or rice from the burner and, once again, very slowly whisk the yolk mixture back into the saucepan combining well, until thickened. Serve immediately.

EXCHANGES/CHOICES 1 Starch | 1 Vegetable | 1/2 Fat

Calories 130 | Calories from Fat 25 | Total Fat 3.0 g | Saturated Fat 1.0 g | Trans Fat 0.0 g
Cholesterol 115 mg | Sodium 150 mg | Potassium 195 mg | Total Carbohydrate 22 g
Dietary Fiber 1 g | Sugars 3 g | Protein 3 g | Phosphorus 145 mg

tortilla soup **with black beans and chilies**

 12 servings

 1/12 recipe

Packed with flavor, fiber, and protein, a bowl of this soup goes a long way. Try using canned chopped tomatoes packed with green chili peppers, for extra flavor.

2 teaspoons olive oil

1 medium red onion, chopped

1/2 medium green bell pepper, cored, seeded, and chopped

1/2 red bell pepper, cored, seeded, and chopped

1 jalapeño pepper, seeded and minced

1 teaspoon ground cumin

2 teaspoons chili powder

1 teaspoon dried leaf oregano

1 cup frozen corn kernels

1 (15-ounce) can black beans, drained and rinsed

2 quarts water or vegetable broth

2 (14-ounce) cans chopped tomatoes packed in juice

1 cup tomato puree

1 pound firm or extra-firm tofu, drained and chopped

1 cup minced cilantro

Juice of 1 lime

2 cups crushed baked tortilla chips

1 Heat the oil in a nonreactive large pot (at least 1 gallon) over medium heat. Add the onions, bell peppers, jalapeños, cumin, chili powder, and oregano. Sauté 3 minutes until onions are lightly browned.

2 Add the corn, black beans, water or broth, tomatoes with their juice, and tomato puree. Bring to a simmer and cook 40 minutes.

3 Add the tofu, cilantro, and lime juice. Stir to combine and heat through. Turn off the heat, add the crushed tortilla chips, and let sit 10 minutes before serving. (If not serving all the soup at one time, only add a portion of the tortilla chips to the soup you are serving immediately.)

EXCHANGES/CHOICES 1 Starch | 1 Vegetable | 1/2 Fat

Calories 130 | Calories from Fat 25 | Total Fat 3.0 g | Saturated Fat 0.4 g | Trans Fat 0.0 g
Cholesterol 0 mg | Sodium 200 mg | Potassium 445 mg | Total Carbohydrate 22 g
Dietary Fiber 5 g | Sugars 5 g | Protein 7 g | Phosphorus 130 mg

white gazpacho with marcona almonds and grapes

 8 servings

 1/8 recipe

Marcona almonds from Spain are rich and aromatic and make this chilled soup refreshing on a warm summer day. If you can't find Marconas, any other unsalted blanched almond will work great.

6 slices white bread, crusts removed

1 cup water plus more to soak the bread, divided use

1 cup unsalted blanched almonds, plus 2 tablespoons chopped almonds (for garnish)

2 cups whole green seedless grapes plus 1/4 cup sliced green grapes (for garnish)

1 cup peeled, seeded, and chopped cucumbers

2 cloves garlic

1 cup fat-free plain yogurt

1/4 cup extra virgin olive oil

1/4 cup sherry vinegar

Salt, to taste

Freshly ground black pepper, to taste

1 Soak the white bread in water for 5 minutes. Drain.

2 Place whole almonds, whole grapes, cucumbers, garlic, and soaked bread in a food processor fitted with the metal blade or a blender. Process or purée until combined. Add the yogurt, 1 cup water, oil, vinegar, salt, and pepper and continue to blend or process until smooth and creamy.

3 Chill at least 30 minutes before serving. Garnish with chopped almonds and sliced grapes.

EXCHANGES/CHOICES 1 1/2 Carbohydrate | 1 Lean Meat | 2 1/2 Fat

Calories 260 | Calories from Fat 155 | Total Fat 17.0 g | Saturated Fat 1.8 g
Trans Fat 0.0 g | Cholesterol 0 mg | Sodium 115 mg | Potassium 330 mg
Total Carbohydrate 22 g | Dietary Fiber 3 g | Sugars 10 g | Protein 7 g
Phosphorus 170 mg

herbed spaetzel and lentil soup

 6 servings

 1 1/2 cups

I learned to make this soup in Germany when I worked for a large hotel. I will always remember making spaetzle the old-fashioned way, for 2,000 people, by hand.

1 tablespoon canola oil

1 large onion, chopped fine

2 medium carrots, peeled and chopped medium

2 stalks celery, chopped medium

3 medium garlic cloves, minced

1 bay leaf

1 teaspoon minced fresh thyme leaves

1 cup lentils, rinsed and picked over for small stones

6 cups water or low-sodium vegetable stock

Salt, to taste

Black pepper, to taste

3 tablespoons minced fresh parsley leaves

1/2 cup spaetzle (page 18)

1 Heat the oil in a large soup pot over medium heat. Add the onions, carrots, celery, garlic, bay leaf, and thyme.

2 Sauté for 2 minutes and add the lentils and stock.

3 Bring to a boil, lower to a simmer, and cook for 45 minutes until lentils are tender. Season with salt and pepper and add the parsley. Add the cooked spaetzle from page 18 for a heartwarming and delicious meal. Discard bay leaf.

EXCHANGES/CHOICES 2 Starch | 1 Vegetable | 1 Lean Meat | 1/2 Fat

Calories 250 | Calories from Fat 45 | Total Fat 5.0 g | Saturated Fat 0.8 g | Trans Fat 0.0 g
Cholesterol 45 mg | Sodium 150 mg | Potassium 640 mg | Total Carbohydrate 39 g
Dietary Fiber 11 g | Sugars 5 g | Protein 14 g | Phosphorus 280 mg

herbed spaetzel

 12 servings

 1/2 cup

This basic recipe for spaetzle can be made with half whole-wheat flour and half unbleached all-purpose flour if you wish. The traditional way to make spaetzle is to use a spaetzle press—which is like a potato ricer—or cut them with a spatula over a cutting board. I offer a much simpler way to make them here. You may add any chopped herb to the batter like dill, basil, or parsley.

1/2 cup 2% milk

1 teaspoon salt

6 large eggs

2 cups whole-wheat flour

1 cup all-purpose white flour

1 tablespoon olive or canola oil

1/4 cup chopped parsley

Salt, to taste

Freshly ground pepper, to taste

Pinch nutmeg

1 In a large mixing bowl combine milk, salt, and eggs with a wire whisk. By hand or with a wooden spoon, gradually add the flour and mix it in. (I always mix with my hand so I can feel the consistency, which should feel like thick pancake batter.)

2 Once the flour is combined, add the oil, parsley, salt, pepper, and nutmeg. Allow mixture to rest for 15 minutes in the bowl.

3 The easiest way to make spaetzle is to place a colander over a large pot of boiling water. Press the spaetzle batter through the colander holes into the water and boil for 3–4 minutes until they float to the top. Immediately transfer the cooked dumplings to a bowl of ice water to cool.

4 Once they are cooled, spray nonstick pan with vegetable or olive oil and sauté spaetzle until heated through. Serve as a side dish, toss with cooked vegetables, or add to soup broth or stock.

EXCHANGES/CHOICES 1 1/2 Starch | 1 Lean Meat

Calories 155 | Calories from Fat 35 | Total Fat 4.0 g | Saturated Fat 1.1 g | Trans Fat 0.0 g
Cholesterol 95 mg | Sodium 235 mg | Potassium 150 mg | Total Carbohydrate 23 g
Dietary Fiber 3 g | Sugars 1 g | Protein 7 g | Phosphorus 140 mg

lots of vegetable soup

 8 servings

 1/8 recipe

Like a liquid garden, full of flavor and texture, this vegetable soup will satisfy even the heartiest appetite.

2 teaspoons canola oil

1 cup chopped onions

1/2 cup chopped celery

1/2 cup diced carrots

1 cup peeled, diced sweet potatoes (1/2-inch dice)

1 cup peeled, diced parsnips (1/2-inch dice)

1 tablespoon minced, peeled gingerroot

2 cloves garlic, minced

3 sprigs fresh thyme

2 bay leaves

2 quarts water

1 teaspoon freshly ground black pepper

1 teaspoon kosher salt

1/2 cup minced fresh dill

1 Heat oil in a saucepan or Dutch oven large enough to hold all ingredients, and sauté vegetables, ginger, and garlic 2 minutes or until lightly browned.

2 Add thyme, bay leaves, and water. Bring to a boil, immediately reduce heat, and simmer 45 minutes until vegetables are tender; do not let boil again. Add pepper, salt, and dill. Remove bay leaves and thyme sprigs before serving.

EXCHANGES/CHOICES 2 Vegetable

Calories 50 | Calories from Fat 15 | Total Fat 1.5 g | Saturated Fat 0.1 g | Trans Fat 0.0 g
Cholesterol 0 mg | Sodium 270 mg | Potassium 185 mg | Total Carbohydrate 9 g
Dietary Fiber 2 g | Sugars 3 g | Protein 1 g | Phosphorus 30 mg

green velvet chilled avocado soup

 4 servings

 1/4 recipe

Wow! I usually hear this twice, first when this luscious jade green soup is placed in front of my guests and then after they taste the first spoonful.

2 ripe avocados, peeled

1 1/2 cups low-sodium vegetable broth, warmed to room temperature

1 (4-ounce) can or jar green chilies, chopped

1/2 cup fat-free plain Greek yogurt

6 scallions, white end trimmed off

1 tablespoon lemon or lime juice

2 teaspoons dry sherry

GARNISH: Chopped canned chilies, fresh cilantro, or crushed tortilla chips

1 Cut the avocados in half and remove the pits. Spoon the avocado into a blender and add all the remaining ingredients (except garnish) and puree until creamy. You may chill the soup for up to 2 hours before serving, or serve immediately.

 CHEF STEVE'S TIPS:

What Are Avocados?
Avocados are a fruit, not a vegetable, which contain 60% more potassium than bananas and about 5 grams of beneficial monounsaturated fat.

To Ripen Avocados:
Place them in a brown paper bag for a few days. If you want to accelerate the process place a banana or apple in the bag with them. The fruit gives off ethylene gas, a ripening agent. You can refrigerate the ripe fruit but only for a day or two.

EXCHANGES/CHOICES 1/2 Carbohydrate | 2 1/2 Fat

Calories 160 | Calories from Fat 100 | Total Fat 11.0 g | Saturated Fat 1.6 g
Trans Fat 0.0 g | Cholesterol 0 mg | Sodium 140 mg | Potassium 535 mg
Total Carbohydrate 12 g | Dietary Fiber 6 g | Sugars 3 g | Protein 5 g
Phosphorus 115 mg

creamy white bean soup
with basil and olive oil

 6 servings

 1/6 recipe

White bean soup is a Tuscan classic. This creamy white bean soup is a perfect backdrop for the beautiful jade green color and perfume of chopped basil. Use jarred white beans for this recipe if available—they are superior to canned.

1 tablespoon extra virgin olive oil

1/2 medium onion, chopped

2 cloves garlic, minced

1 ripe tomato, chopped

2 teaspoons dried oregano

Pinch of crushed red chili flakes

1 (20-ounce) jar of white beans with liquid or an equivalent amount of canned white beans, drained and rinsed

4 cups low-sodium vegetable broth

6–8 fresh basil leaves, minced

Juice of 1 fresh lemon

Sea salt, to taste

1 Heat oil in a large saucepot over medium heat. Sauté the onion and garlic for 1 minute, stirring often.

2 Add the tomato, oregano, and crushed chili flakes. Continue to sauté for another minute. Add the beans and broth. Bring to a boil, lower to a simmer, and cook uncovered for 35 minutes until smooth and creamy.

3 Add the basil and lemon juice, season to taste with salt.

 CHEF STEVE'S TIP:

Make simple garlic-Parmesan croutons for the soup by slicing French bread into thin rounds, rubbing with garlic cloves, and brushing with extra virgin olive oil. Sprinkle Parmesan cheese over the rounds. Bake on a pan in a 375°F oven for 5–7 minutes until golden brown. Serve with soup.

EXCHANGES/CHOICES 1 Starch | 1 Lean Meat

Calories 115 | Calories from Fat 20 | Total Fat 2.5 g | Saturated Fat 0.4 g | Trans Fat 0.0 g
Cholesterol 0 mg | Sodium 200 mg | Potassium 425 mg | Total Carbohydrate 18 g
Dietary Fiber 6 g | Sugars 4 g | Protein 5 g | Phosphorus 165 mg

chicpea and hominy stew

 6 servings

 8 ounces

Hominy is so misunderstood. This stew is the perfect introduction to these cooked kernels of corn with their sweet, nutty, and aromatic flavor. Keep a can or two on your pantry shelves to liven up any soup or stew.

2 teaspoons canola, olive, or corn oil

2 cups onion, diced

3 cloves garlic, minced

1 poblano or Anaheim chili, minced

2 (19-ounce) cans cooked chickpeas, drained and rinsed

1 (19-ounce) can cooked hominy, drained and rinsed

1 large tomato, diced

Water or vegetable stock to barely cover

2 cups fresh kale or spinach, coarsely chopped

1/2 teaspoon kosher salt

1/4 teaspoon black pepper

1 Heat the oil over medium-high heat in a large saucepan. Sauté the onion, garlic, and poblano or Anaheim chili for 1 minute.

2 Add the chickpeas, hominy, and tomato and barely cover with water or stock. Bring to a boil, lower to a simmer, and cook covered for 20 minutes.

3 Add the chopped greens, simmer for 1 minute longer, and season with salt and pepper.

EXCHANGES/CHOICES 2 Starch | 2 Vegetable | 1 Lean Meat | 1/2 Fat

Calories 275 | Calories from Fat 45 | Total Fat 5.0 g | Saturated Fat 0.5 g | Trans Fat 0.0 g
Cholesterol 0 mg | Sodium 440 mg | Potassium 605 mg | Total Carbohydrate 48 g
Dietary Fiber 12 g | Sugars 12 g | Protein 12 g | Phosphorus 240 mg

five alarm garden chili

 12 servings

 8 ounces

This is a hearty, spicy, comforting chili thickened with cracked wheat. It is also extremely forgiving because you can add any fresh-cut vegetable to the recipe. For a gluten-free version, replace the cracked wheat with barley or quinoa. Chipotle chilis en adobo are smoked dried jalapeños in a tomato sauce. They are available in small cans in the ethnic section of most supermarkets.

1 tablespoon olive oil

1 1/2 cups onion, chopped

1 cup carrot, chopped

1 cup celery, chopped

1 cup red pepper, chopped

1 cup mushrooms, chopped

2 jalapeño peppers, seeds removed, and minced

1 canned chipotle chili en adobo, minced

1 cup bulgur wheat (cracked wheat)

2 teaspoons oregano, dry

1 teaspoon cumin seed, ground

1 1/2 teaspoons chili powder

1 1/2 teaspoons cocoa powder, unsweetened

1 (28-ounce) can low-sodium crushed tomatoes

3 cups water

1 (16-ounce) can kidney or pinto beans

2 tablespoons fresh cilantro, minced

2 tablespoons lime juice

GARNISH: Plain low-fat yogurt, grated low-fat cheddar cheese, and minced red onion (optional)

1 In a large saucepot heat olive oil over moderate heat. Add onion, carrot, celery, red pepper, mushrooms, jalapeños, chili en adobo, and bulgur. Sauté for 3 minutes and add oregano, cumin seed, chili powder, and cocoa powder and continue to sauté for another minute.

2 Add crushed tomatoes, water, and cooked beans and simmer for 40 minutes slowly until wheat becomes tender and sauce thickens.

3 Add cilantro and lime. Garnish with plain, fat-free yogurt, a sprinkling of cheddar, and some minced red onion, if desired.

EXCHANGES/CHOICES 1 Starch | 1 Vegetable | 1/2 Fat

Calories 130 | Calories from Fat 20 | Total Fat 2.0 g | Saturated Fat 0.3 g | Trans Fat 0.0 g
Cholesterol 0 mg | Sodium 145 mg | Potassium 495 mg | Total Carbohydrate 23 g
Dietary Fiber 6 g | Sugars 5 g | Protein 6 g | Phosphorus 125 mg

lentil dal

 6 servings

 1/6 recipe

This version of Indian dal is chunkier and thinner than a typical dal. It has whole identifiable vegetables in it, making it filling and satisfying.

1 tablespoon olive oil

1 cup chopped onions

4 cloves garlic, minced

1 tablespoon minced ginger

1 teaspoon cumin seeds

1/2 teaspoon crushed red chili flakes

1 teaspoon turmeric

2 cups chopped tomato (2 medium fresh, or canned)

2 cups chopped cauliflower

1 cup brown or green lentils (red may be used; however, sauce will be thinner)

2 1/2 cups water or vegetable broth

1 teaspoon salt

1/8 cup lime juice

6 sprigs minced cilantro

1 Heat oil in a 2 1/2-quart saucepot and sauté onions, garlic, ginger, and spices for 2 minutes.

2 Add tomatoes and cauliflower and sauté 1 minute longer.

3 Add the lentils and combine well. Pour the liquid over the lentils, bring to a boil, cover, and simmer slowly for 35–40 minutes until vegetables and lentils are tender.

4 Season with salt, lime, and cilantro. Serve over basmati or jasmine rice.

EXCHANGES/CHOICES 1 Starch | 1 Vegetable | 1 Lean Meat

Calories 160 | Calories from Fat 25 | Total Fat 3.0 g | Saturated Fa 0.4 g | Trans Fat 0.0 g
Cholesterol 0 mg | Sodium 405 mg | Potassium 660 mg | Total Carbohydrate 26 g
Dietary Fiber 9 g | Sugars 5 g | Protein 10 g | Phosphorus 205 mg

miso-noodle soup

 8 servings

 8 ounces

Miso is a staple in Japan. It's complex in flavor with a sweet, salty wine-like taste. It comes in several varieties with white miso being the mildest. Dark brown or red miso is more pungent and aged longer. Full of active enzymes, it is a living product best added at the end of a cooking process to preserve its nutritional properties.

4 ounces noodles, dry (angel hair, Chinese egg noodles, or Udon)

2 teaspoons canola or olive oil

1 teaspoon sesame oil, dark roasted

2 cloves garlic, minced

1 teaspoon grated gingerroot

1 teaspoon chili paste (Thai or Chinese)

6 cups low-sodium vegetable broth or water

2 cups broccoli florets

1 cup carrots, sliced on the bias

1 cup onion, sliced thinly

1/4 cup white miso

6 scallions, sliced thinly

1/2 cup bean sprouts

1/2 teaspoon Chinese five-spice powder (optional)

1 Cook the noodles in boiling water until tender, rinse in cold water, and set aside.

2 Heat both oils in a saucepan over medium heat. Add the garlic and ginger and sauté for 1 minute. Add the chili paste.

3 Add the water or broth, bring to a boil, and add all the vegetable. Simmer the vegetables for 2 minutes until almost tender.

4 Add the cooked noodles, miso, scallions, and bean sprouts.

EXCHANGES/CHOICES 1 Starch | 1 Vegetable | 1/2 Fat

Calories 115 | Calories from Fat 20 | Total Fat 2.5 g | Saturated Fat 0.2 g | Trans Fat 0.0 g
Cholesterol 0 mg | Sodium 295 mg | Potassium 295 mg | Total Carbohydrate 20 g
Dietary Fiber 3 g | Sugars 6 g | Protein 3 g | Phosphorus 120 mg

pasta con fagioli

 10 servings

 8 ounces

I like to leave this soup thick and chunky; however, it is often puréed to a smooth consistency. I also alter the classical version by adding just a little tomato paste, which adds a little tartness and color. My chef's secret is to cook the pasta separately and add it at the end to keep it al dente.

1/2 cup cavatelli or orechiette pasta, uncooked

1 tablespoon olive oil

4 cloves garlic, minced

1 cup minced red onion

1 cup chopped celery

2 teaspoons dried Italian herbs

1/2 teaspoon red chili flakes

2 bay leaves

1 medium tomato, chopped

1/2 cup marinara sauce

2 (15 ounce) cans cannellini beans, drained and rinsed well

6–7 cups water or vegetable broth

2 cups coarsely chopped Swiss chard or spinach

1 teaspoon salt

1 Cook pasta al dente according to directions. Drain and set aside.

2 Heat oil in a 5 1/2-quart saucepot. Sauté garlic, red onion, celery, herbs, chili flakes, bay leaves, and tomato for 3 minutes, then add marinara sauce and beans. Cover with water and bring to a boil. Lower to a simmer and cook for 35–40 minutes until all ingredients are tender and combined well.

3 Add chard or spinach and cooked pasta. Simmer for 5 minutes longer and season with salt. Add additional water or broth if soup becomes too thick. Remove bay leaves before serving.

EXCHANGES/CHOICES 1 Starch | 1 Vegetable | 1/2 Fat

Calories 115 | Calories from Fat 20 | Total Fat 2.0 g | Saturated Fat 0.3 g | Trans Fat 0.0 g
Cholesterol 0 mg | Sodium 365 mg | Potassium 365 mg | Total Carbohydrate 20 g
Dietary Fiber 4 g | Sugars 3 g | Protein 6 g | Phosphorus 95 mg

CHAPTER 2
Raw and Ready Salads

There is nothing like a well-constructed salad because the components are the star attraction. I can remember when salad meant a wedge of iceberg lettuce with a slice of tomato and maybe a cucumber or onion ring perched up on that huge wedge. Greens are only the beginning when it comes to a great salad and we are fortunate to have so many varieties available year round. Most groceries stock fresh baby arugula, watercress, tat soi, and red endives.

Another important salad component is selecting the right cheese. Crisp endive slices, ripe sweet pear, and toasted walnuts would be missing something without a good stilton or blue cheese. Minted chickpeas would protest if it were not for a topping of creamy feta cheese.

The salads in this chapter are all about the juxtaposition of unlikely ingredients and how they relate to your palate. Thoughtfully combining textures that might not normally get along like crispy or crunchy foods against the soft and silky background of a seasonal vegetable. The pleasant and welcome conflict of a warm roasted beet pitted against chilled Greek yogurt, or the clash of fresh grapefruit against creamy delicate avocado. When you add a drizzle of homemade dressing or fine olive oil everything seems to harmonize nicely in your mouth at the very same moment. Perfect culinary partners without the application of heat, who would have thought?

endive salad **with stilton, pear, and walnuts**

 4 servings

 1/4 recipe

There is a reason why the combination of Stilton, pear, and walnuts are considered classic. One taste explains this without words. Pungent Stilton or blue cheese is perfect with slightly bitter endives and sweet ripe pears. The walnuts add a rich pleasant bonus.

2 heads endive, thinly sliced crosswise into rounds

3 tablespoons crumbled Stilton, blue, or gorgonzola cheese

1/4 cup chopped walnuts

1 ripe pear, halved, cored, and sliced thinly crosswise

1 tablespoon extra-virgin olive oil

Juice of 1/2 lemon

Kosher salt, to taste

Freshly ground black pepper, to taste

1 Combine all ingredients in a medium bowl and toss.

 CHEF STEVE'S TIPS:

Walnuts are a nutrient-dense food packed with flavor. Being of Russian descent, I remember my grandparents using walnuts after keeping them in the freezer. This keeps walnuts fresher for longer.

EXCHANGES/CHOICES 1/2 Fruit | 1 Vegetable | 2 Fat

Calories 155 | Calories from Fat 90 | Total Fat 10.0 g | Saturated Fat 2.2 g | Trans Fat 0.1 g
Cholesterol 5 mg | Sodium 120 mg | Potassium 565 mg | Total Carbohydrate 13 g
Dietary Fiber 6 g | Sugars 5 g | Protein 5 g | Phosphorus 95 mg

luscious avocado-strawberry salad with toasted pine nuts

 4 servings

 1/4 recipe

Worthy of a special occasion, yet incredibly simple. This is one of my all-time favorites. Try papaya or mango in season in place of the strawberries.

1 ripe avocado, preferably Hass variety, peeled, pitted, and cut into chunks

Juice of 1 lemon or lime

1 heaping cup strawberries, hulled and cut into 1/2-inch-thick slices

1 tablespoon extra virgin olive oil, walnut oil, or hazelnut oil

2 tablespoons raspberry vinegar

2 teaspoons honey

Salt, to taste

Freshly ground black pepper, to taste

2 cups bite-sized pieces arugula or watercress

2 tablespoons toasted pine nuts

1 Combine avocado with lemon juice in a nonreactive large bowl. Add berries, oil, vinegar, honey, salt, and pepper and combine well. Serve over a bed of arugula or watercress on each of the four plates. Garnish with pine nuts.

 CHEF STEVE'S TIPS:

To toast pine nuts: Place in a dry sauté pan or skillet over medium heat 3–4 minutes, stirring often, until they begin to brown.

EXCHANGES/CHOICES 1 Carbohydrate | 2 Fat

Calories 160 | Calories from Fat 110 | Total Fat 12.0 g | Saturated Fat 1.5 g
Trans Fat 0.0 g | Cholesterol 0 mg | Sodium 10 mg | Potassium 340 mg
Total Carbohydrate 14 g | Dietary Fiber 4 g | Sugars 8 g | Protein 2 g | Phosphorus 65 mg

terra cotta **cobb salad**

 4 servings

 1/4 recipe

This Southwestern version of the classic Cobb has it all going on. Colorful, crunchy, spicy, tart, and fulfilling, it can be served as a complete meal. Roasted bite-sized tofu can be added for additional protein.

1 (5-ounce) bag of field greens, baby spinach, or arugula

1/2 cup red pepper, chopped

1/2 cup green pepper, chopped

1/2 cup red onion, chopped

1/2 cup tomato, chopped

1 avocado, diced

1 cup fat-free shredded cheddar cheese

1 cup canned black beans, drained and rinsed well

1/4 cup shelled pumpkin seeds

4 tablespoons Lime Drizzle

1 Place the field greens on a large serving platter. Arrange all the chopped vegetables, cheese, and black beans in colorful rows across the greens.

2 Sprinkle the shelled pumpkin seeds on top and drizzle with dressing.

LIME DRIZZLE

 4 servings

 1–2 tablespoons

1/4 cup extra virgin olive oil

1/4 cup lime juice

2 teaspoons honey

2 tablespoons minced cilantro

1 Combine all ingredients well in a small mixing bowl with a wire whisk or blend with a hand-held immersion blender until smooth.

EXCHANGES/CHOICES (includes Lime Drizzle) 1 Starch | 1 Vegetable | 2 Lean Meat 2 1/2 Fat

Calories 300 | Calories from Fat 145 | Total Fat 16.0 g | Saturated Fat 2.5 g
Trans Fat 0.0 g | Cholesterol 5 mg | Sodium 350 mg | Potassium 660 mg
Total Carbohydrate 23 g | Dietary Fiber 9 g | Sugars 6 g | Protein 17 g
Phosphorus 335 mg

tofu niçoise salad

 4 servings

 1/4 recipe

Tofu takes on the role of traditional tuna in this classic French salad served throughout southern France. This entrée salad has tons of texture and flavor.

LEMON DRESSING

1/4 cup very good-quality Spanish, Italian, or Greek extra virgin olive oil

Juice of 2 lemons

2 teaspoons Dijon mustard

2 tablespoons chopped parsley

NIÇOISE SALAD

1 pound firm tofu, cut into 1/2-inch slices

Water

Salt, to taste

3/4 pound fresh green beans, cut into 2-inch lengths

3 cups bite-sized pieces salad greens or field greens

1 medium tomato, cut into wedges

2 hard-boiled eggs, sliced or cut into wedges

1 cup cooked dried chickpeas or drained and rinsed canned chickpeas

1 small red onion, sliced into 1/4-inch rings

1/4 cup kalamata olives

2 tablespoons drained and rinsed capers

1. Combine all dressing ingredients in a nonreactive container and whisk to combine.

2. Lay tofu slices in a single layer in a nonreactive dish. Coat with 2 tablespoons dressing and let marinate 1 hour. (This can be done up to 2 days prior to use.) Preheat a charcoal or gas grill or oven broiler element. Grill marinated tofu 3 minutes on each side or broil 2 inches from heating element 5 minutes per side. Set aside to cool. Cut into fingers or bite-sized squares. Set aside.

3. Bring a saucepan of lightly salted water to boil over high heat. Add green beans and boil 3 minutes or until bright green yet still crisp. Drain and rinse under cold water.

4. Place lettuce on a serving platter. Arrange all ingredients: beans, tofu, tomato, eggs, chickpeas, onions, olives, and capers decoratively over the greens and drizzle with remaining dressing.

EXCHANGES/CHOICES 1/2 Starch | 3 Vegetable | 2 Med-Fat Meat | 3 Fat

Calories 390 | Calories from Fat 225 | Total Fat 25.0 g | Saturated Fat 4.1 g
Trans Fat 0.0 g | Cholesterol 95 mg | Sodium 390 mg | Potassium 660 mg
Total Carbohydrate 27 g | Dietary Fibe 9 g | Sugars 7 g | Protein 19 g
Phosphorus 305 mg

roasted beet salad with skordalia (potato dip)

 6 servings

 1/6 recipe

This contemporary version of an ancient recipe pairs sweet roasted beets with creamy potato dip. Perfect as an appetizer or salad course, this is a great way to start any meal.

2 medium red beets, peeled and cut into small wedges

2 medium golden beets, peeled and cut into small wedges

2 teaspoons olive oil

1/8 teaspoon cinnamon

Salt, to taste

Freshly ground black pepper, to taste

1 cup plus 2 tablespoons skordalia (Potato Dip, page 132), divided use

3 cups field greens

1   Preheat oven to 375°F.

2   In a medium bowl, toss beets, oil, cinnamon, salt, and pepper. Place on a baking pan with sides and bake 35–40 minutes until just tender and lightly browned. Set aside.

3   Place 3 tablespoons skordalia in the center of each of 6 plates. Scatter 1/2 cup field greens around the plate. Top skordalia with a few pieces of roasted beets and serve.

EXCHANGES/CHOICES 1/2 Starch | 1 Vegetable | 1 1/2 Fat

Calories 140 | Calories from Fat 70 | Total Fat 8.0 g | Saturated Fat 1.2 g | Trans Fat 0.0 g
Cholesterol 0 mg | Sodium 165 mg | Potassium 380 mg | Total Carbohydrate 15 g
Dietary Fiber 2 g | Sugars 4 g | Protein 2 g | Phosphorus 45 mg

minted chickpeas and feta with kalamata olives

 10 servings

 1/10 recipe

Smoked paprika gives this salad a warm ruby color and smoky flavor that combines well with pungent feta and cooling mint. You can mix this salad with couscous or serve over a bed of cooked couscous as an entrée.

4 cups canned chickpeas, drained and rinsed well

1 medium tomato, chopped

1/4 cup minced red onions

1/4 cup chopped pitted kalamata olives

2 tablespoons extra virgin olive oil

1 tablespoon red wine vinegar

1 tablespoon lemon juice

2 teaspoons smoked paprika

1/3 cup crumbled reduced-fat feta cheese

1/4 cup chopped parsley

1/4 cup chopped fresh mint

Freshly ground black pepper, to taste

4 cups field greens or 6 lettuce leaves (optional)

1 Combine all ingredients except lettuce in a large mixing bowl and toss with a spoon. Let marinate 15 minutes or refrigerate overnight. Serve as is, or over a bed of lettuce leaves or field greens.

EXCHANGES/CHOICES 1 Starch | 1 Lean Meat | 1/2 Fat

Calories 155 | Calories from Fat 55 | Total Fat 6.0 g | Saturated Fat 1.0 g | Trans Fat 0.0 g | Cholesterol 0 mg | Sodium 220 mg | Potassium 245 mg | Total Carbohydrate 19 g | Dietary Fiber 5 g | Sugars 4 g | Protein 7 g | Phosphorus 125 mg

singapore cucumber salad

 4 servings

 1/4 recipe

Seedless mini cucumbers are cropping up everywhere lately. They are also called Persian cucumbers. Feel free to substitute Kirby cucumbers in the same quantity. Mirin (rice wine), Sriracha sauce, and sambal oelek or chili paste with garlic can be found in Asian markets and some supermarkets. This is a great salad or sandwich topping as well.

6 mini seedless cucumbers or 1 large seedless cucumber, thinly sliced on the bias

12 red, yellow, or orange mini-bell peppers, cored, seeded, and thinly sliced, or 1 each yellow and red bell pepper, cored, seeded, and thinly sliced

1/2 cup thin-sliced red onions

1 navel orange, peeled, halved, and thinly sliced

1 tablespoon reduced-sodium soy sauce or tamari

2 tablespoons Mirin

1 tablespoon unseasoned rice vinegar

1 teaspoon Sriracha sauce or sambal oelek (chili paste with garlic)

2 teaspoons brown or black sesame seeds

1 Combine all ingredients in a large mixing bowl and allow to sit 10 minutes before serving.

 CHEF STEVE'S TIP:

Sriracha is my new ketchup. It's spicy and lends itself to so many dishes, from scrambled eggs to soup, stews, and salads. I always have a bottle in my refrigerator.

EXCHANGES/CHOICES 1/2 Fruit | 1 Vegetable

Calories 70 | Calories from Fat 10 | Total Fat 1.0 g | Saturated Fat 0.2 g | Trans Fat 0.0 g
Cholesterol 0 mg | Sodium 165 mg | Potassium 320 mg | Total Carbohydrate 13 g
Dietary Fiber 2 g | Sugars 7 g | Protein 2 g | Phosphorus 60 mg

watercress, golden beets, and fennel salad **with parmesan-peppercorn dressing**

 6 servings

 1/6 recipe

A kaleidoscope of color, texture, and taste, this salad is so simple, yet incredibly complex in its flavor profile. It can literally be made in minutes. Sunchokes, also called Jerusalem artichokes, are crunchy, sweet, and can be eaten raw or cooked. If you can't find sunchokes, use jicama, also a sweet root vegetable.

PARMESAN-PEPPERCORN DRESSING

1/2 cup fat-free Greek-style yogurt

3/4 cup low-fat buttermilk

2 cloves garlic

1/4 cup minced fresh dill

1/2 cup freshly grated parmesan cheese

1/8 cup apple cider vinegar

1 tablespoon freshly ground black pepper

SALAD

1 small head Boston or butter lettuce, separated into leaves

2 golden beets, peeled and grated or cut into matchsticks

2 large sunchokes, peeled and thinly sliced

1 medium fennel (anise) bulb, trimmed and thinly sliced

1 bunch watercress, heavy ends trimmed (about 1 1/2 cups)

1 Combine all dressing ingredients in a food processor fitted with the metal blade or a blender. Process or purée until smooth. Set aside.

2 Wash and pat dry all of the salad greens. Arrange lettuce leaves to cover a large plate or bowl.

3 In a large mixing bowl, combine the beets, sunchokes, fennel, and watercress and toss lightly.

4 Toss the vegetables with the dressing or drizzle it on at the end. Place the vegetables on the prepared plate or in the bowl. Drizzle with dressing if you didn't toss it with the vegetables.

EXCHANGES/CHOICES 1/2 Starch | 2 Vegetable | 1/2 Fat

Calories 105 | Calories from Fat 20 | Total Fat 2.0 g | Saturated Fat 1.2 g | Trans Fat 0.0 g
Cholesterol 5 mg | Sodium 185 mg | Potassium 625 mg | Total Carbohydrate 16 g
Dietary Fiber 3 g | Sugars 8 g | Protein 8 g | Phosphorus 175 mg

radish and cucumber salad
with gorgonzola cheese

 4 servings

 1/4 recipe

So simple to prepare, this recipe is deceiving. When these few ingredients combine, they burst with flavor, texture, and antioxidants. Great for a family dinner, but elegant enough for company.

8 medium radishes, thinly sliced

1/3 English cucumbers, thinly sliced

3 scallions, thinly sliced

2 tablespoons crumbled Gorgonzola cheese

2 tablespoons rice vinegar

1 tablespoon extra virgin olive oil

2 tablespoons walnuts, chopped

Salt and pepper, to taste

1 Combine all ingredients in a medium bowl and serve.

 CHEF STEVE'S TIP:

Try feta, blue, or Manchego cheese as an alternative to Gorgonzola.

EXCHANGES/CHOICES 1 Vegetable | 1 1/2 Fat

Calories 80 | Calories from Fat 65 | Total Fat 7.0 g | Saturated Fat 1.5 g | Trans Fat 0.0 g
Cholesterol 5 mg | Sodium 65 mg | Potassium 135 mg | Total Carbohydrate 3 g
Dietary Fiber 1 g | Sugars 1g | Protein 2 g | Phosphorus 45 mg

barley and corn strata salad in mason jars

 6 servings

 1/6 recipe

What a great way to impress your friends and family. Serve this salad in layers in an old-fashioned mason jar.

1 cup pearled barley

2 1/2 cups water or vegetable or chicken stock

1 teaspoon grated lemon peel

1 stalk celery, sliced

1 cup frozen or fresh corn

1 carrot, grated

1/4 cup frozen peas

1 teaspoon salt

LAYERS

1/2 cup grape tomatoes, halved

1 cup chopped fresh spinach leaves

1/2 cup sliced button mushrooms

1 Add pearl barley to water or stock. Bring to a boil, lower to a simmer, and cover. Add lemon zest and simmer for approximately 35–40 minutes. Allow to rest for 10 minutes then transfer to a bowl, fluff with a fork and cool slightly.

2 Add celery, corn, carrot, and peas. Season with salt and cool completely before layering in jars.

3 Place a layer of barley salad on bottom of jar. Arrange half the tomatoes over salad. Arrange half the spinach, then half the mushrooms, and another layer of barley salad. Repeat process forming 2 layers of ingredients.

EXCHANGES/CHOICES 2 Starch

Calories 150 | Calories from Fat 5 | Total Fat 0.5 g | Saturated Fat 0.1 g | Trans Fat 0.0 g
Cholesterol 0 mg | Sodium 420 mg | Potassium 285 mg | Total Carbohydrate 34 g
Dietary Fiber 7 g | Sugars 2 g | Protein 5 g | Phosphorus 110 mg

campfire corn and black bean salad

 6 servings

 1/6 recipe

Sweet, crunchy, spicy, and colorful, this salad is a workhorse and you can serve it over greens, raw spinach, or grilled tofu. It makes a great wrap as well with lettuce, hummus, or a shredded sharp cheddar or Jack cheese.

2 tablespoons olive oil

1/4 cup red onion, diced

1/2 red pepper, diced

1/2 green pepper, diced

1 (15-ounce) can black beans, drained and rinsed

1 (12-ounce) bag frozen roasted corn or regular frozen corn

2 tablespoons lime juice

Salt, to taste

1/4 cup fresh cilantro, minced

1/4 cup chopped canned green chilies (optional)

1   In a large mixing bowl, combine the oil, onion, peppers, beans, corn, lime, salt, and cilantro. Let stand for 20 minutes before serving. Top with the green chilies, if desired.

CHEF STEVE'S TIP:

Cliantro is one of those ingredients that no one sits on the fence about. It is quite pungent, but always unforgettable. You can substitute parsley if you prefer.

EXCHANGES/CHOICES 1 1/2 Starch | 1 Fat

Calories 150 | Calories from Fat 45 | Total Fat 5.0 g | Saturated Fat 0.8 g | Trans Fat 0.0 g
Cholesterol 0 mg | Sodium 55 mg | Potassium 330 mg | Total Carbohydrate 24 g
Dietary Fiber 5 g | Sugars 3 g | Protein 6 g | Phosphorus 105 mg

crunchy cajun **cabbage slaw**

 10 servings

 1/10 recipe

Not your mother's cole slaw, this powerhouse of cruciferous vegetables packs some heat! Perfect as a side dish or heaped on top of a sandwich.

DRESSING

1/2 cup low-fat mayonnaise

1/2 cup fat-free Greek yogurt

1 tablespoon Dijon mustard

3 tablespoons apple cider vinegar

2 tablespoons agave or honey

1 teaspoon sea or kosher salt

1/2 teaspoon black pepper

SLAW VEGETABLES

5 cups green cabbage, sliced thinly

3 cups red cabbage, sliced thinly

4 kale or collard green leaves, heavy stem removed, sliced thinly

2 carrots, peeled and shredded

4 scallions, minced

1 Combine dressing ingredients in a large mixing bowl with a wire whisk.

2 Add vegetables and mix well. Allow to marinate for at least 1 hour before serving.

 CHEF STEVE'S TIP:

Fat-free Greek yogurt is a great substitute for mayonnaise in most every recipe.

EXCHANGES/CHOICES 1/2 Carbohydrate | 1 Vegetable

Calories 65 | Calories from Fat 10 | Total Fat 1.0 g | Saturated Fat 0.2 g | Trans Fat 0.0 g
Cholesterol 0 mg | Sodium 405 mg | Potassium 230 mg | Total Carbohydrate 12 g
Dietary Fiber 3 g | Sugars 7 g | Protein 3 g | Phosphorus 45 mg

sweet potato and apple salad
with chipotle lime dressing

 6 servings

 1/6 recipe

Serve this salad as is or over greens, arugula, or spinach leaves. Sweet potatoes will keep for 3 days in the refrigerator if they are well covered. It makes a killer quesadilla or burrito when combined with a bit of melted cheddar or Monterey Jack cheese.

2 pounds sweet potatoes, peeled and cut into 1-inch dice

1 large apple, such as Fuji, Gala, or Granny Smith, cut into 1/2-inch chunks

1/2 medium red bell pepper, chopped

1/2 green pepper, chopped

1 celery stalk, chopped

1/4 red onion, chopped

2 tablespoons chopped fresh cilantro

CHIPOTLE LIME DRESSING

2 chipotle chilies en adobo

1/4 cup lime juice

1 tablespoon honey or molasses

2 tablespoons tomato catsup

1 clove garlic, peeled

1/4 cup extra virgin olive oil

1 Place the sweet potatoes in boiling, lightly salted water in a large saucepan and boil, covered, for 8–10 minutes until tender. Drain and set aside on a plate.

2 Combine the apple, bell peppers, celery, red onion, and cilantro in a large bowl. Add the cooked potatoes, mixing lightly.

3 Combine all the dressing ingredients, except for the oil, in a food processor and puree together. Drizzle in the oil and continue to process until thick.

4 Add the dressing to the vegetables and toss well.

EXCHANGES/CHOICES 2 1/2 Carbohydrate | 1 1/2 Fat

Calories 235 | Calories from Fat 80 | Total Fat 9.0 g | Saturated Fat 1.3 g | Trans Fat 0.0 g
Cholesterol 0 mg | Sodium 120 mg | Potassium 470 mg | Total Carbohydrate 37 g
Dietary Fiber 5 g | Sugars 17 g | Protein 3 g | Phosphorus 65 mg

grapefruit and avocado salad
with honey mustard citrus dressing

 4 servings

 1/4 recipe

Buttery smooth avocado combines well with tart citrus fruit in this recipe. A drizzle of Honey Mustard Citrus Dressing creates a perfect background for both. Cut the peel away from the citrus fruits using a sharp knife, which removes the bitter white pith of the fruit.

1 medium avocado, halved, peeled, and cut into 1/2-inch chunks

1 pink grapefruit, peeled and cut into sections or wheels

1 navel orange, peeled and cut into sections or wheels

1/2 red pepper, chopped

4 green onions, minced

4 cups field greens or torn romaine

1 Combine all ingredients, except the field greens, in a large nonreactive mixing bowl. Toss with half of the Honey Mustard Citrus Dressing (below) to moisten. Serve over a nest of field greens.

EXCHANGES/CHOICES 1 Fruit | 1 Vegetable | 3 Fat

Calories 235 | Calories from Fat 145 | Total Fat 16.0 g | Saturated Fat 2.3 g
Trans Fat 0.0 g | Cholesterol 0 mg | Sodium 100 mg | Potassium 575 mg
Total Carbohydrate 24 g | Dietary Fiber 6 g | Sugars 15 g | Protein 3 g | Phosphorus 65 mg

HONEY MUSTARD CITRUS DRESSING

 8 servings

 2 tablespoons

1/3 cup orange juice

6 tablespoons extra virgin olive oil

3 tablespoons lime juice

2 tablespoons honey

2 tablespoons Dijon mustard

1 Combine all ingredients in a food processor or blender and process for 1 minute until smooth and creamy. This recipe makes more dressing than you will need to toss salad. You may serve with the extra dressing.

EXCHANGES/CHOICES 1/2 Carbohydrate | 2 Fat

Calories 115 | Calories from Fat 90 | Total Fat 10.0 g
Saturated Fat 1.4 g | Trans Fat 0.0 g | Cholesterol 0 mg
Sodium 90 mg | Potassium 35 mg | Total Carbohydrate 7 g
Dietary Fiber 0 g | Sugars 6 g | Protein 0 g | Phosphorus 5 mg

CHAPTER 3
Hand to Mouth: Burgers, Patties, and Griddlecakes

Burgers, patties, and griddlecakes are the staple of American cooking tradition. We just love any food that we can hold in our hands while we multitask. The burgers presented here in this vegetarian collection are unlike any you have ever had before. They each have a very different character, mouth feel, and bold flavor. These burgers are made with wonderful whole grains, Asian noodles, and antioxidant-rich vegetables. They have little or no cholesterol and are as comforting as any burger that has ever landed between buns.

These burgers can be dressed up as you would any other traditional burger or enjoyed "naked" on the plate. Most of the burger recipes can be made into sliders (mini burgers) or formed into loaf pans and baked "meatloaf" style as well. They can be made in advance up to a few days prior to browning or baking.

You are going to want to dress these burgers up with some of the salsas and sauces you'll also find in this book. Topping a grilled black bean burger with a juicy picnic salsa with ripe seasonal summer fruits is so much more engaging than standard fare. What can be more comforting than a roasted **Eggplant Risotto Cakes** (page 48) topped with **Salsa Minestrone** (page 131)? There are enough burger varieties in this chapter for every taste and preference—you may find that even the carnivores in your life will be delighted with every bite.

feelin' your oats burgers

 12 servings

 1 burger

In this recipe, I have you make a rectangular patty from the oat mixture and then cut it into individual burgers. However, you can shape the burgers by stamping rounds with a glass. Nutritional yeast is available at natural food stores.

4 cups water

1/4 cup reduced-sodium soy sauce or tamari

1 cup chopped onions

1 rib celery, chopped

1 tablespoon dried Italian herb blend (oregano, rosemary, and thyme)

1/4 cup chopped walnuts

2 teaspoons nutritional yeast (optional)

4 1/2 cups rolled oats (not instant oats)

1 Place the water, soy sauce or tamari, onions, celery, herbs, walnuts, and yeast, if using, in a large saucepan.

2 Bring to a boil over high heat. Boil 4 minutes and then add oats. Stirring constantly, simmer 5 minutes until the mixture is the consistency of really thick wet sand.

3 Scoop the mixture into an 11 × 7–inch baking pan. Pat the mixture until it is spread evenly.

4 Preheat oven to 375°F. Place the uncovered pan in the center of the oven and bake about 30 minutes.

5 Remove pan from oven and cool slightly. Keep oven set to 375°F.

6 With a spatula, cut oat mixture into rectangular burgers. Remove burgers to a baking pan with sides and bake another 10 minutes until crisp.

EXCHANGES/CHOICES 1 1/2 Starch | 1/2 Fat

Calories 145 | Calories from Fat 30 | Total Fat 3.5 g | Saturated Fat 0.5 g | Trans Fat 0.0 g | Cholesterol 0 mg | Sodium 190 mg | Potassium 165 mg | Total Carbohydrate 23 g | Dietary Fiber 4 g | Sugars 1 g | Protein 5 g | Phosphorus 145 mg

black bean patties **with cilantro and lime**

 10 servings

 1 (4 oz) patty

Comforting, spicy, and warming on a cool day, these patties take the cake. Wonderful on a whole-grain bun, over a salad, or simply on a plate with sliced onions.

1 tablespoon olive oil

1 cup onion, chopped

1/2 cup green pepper, chopped

1/2 cup red pepper, chopped

1 jalapeño, minced

2 cloves garlic, minced

1 teaspoon chili powder

1/2 teaspoon oregano

1/2 teaspoon ground cumin

1 (16-ounce) can black beans with liquid

1 1/2 cups breadcrumbs, unseasoned

1/2 cup cornmeal, yellow or white

1 tablespoon lime juice

3/4 teaspoon salt

1/4 cup reduced-fat cheddar or Jack cheese

2 tablespoons cilantro, minced

1 In a large nonstick pan heat olive oil and sauté onions, peppers, garlic, and spices. Sauté for 3 minutes, or until vegetables are tender.

2 Add black beans with liquid and sauté with vegetables for 1 minute. Remove from heat. Add breadcrumbs, cornmeal, lime juice, and salt. Remove 1 cup of bean mixture and purée in a blender or food processor until a coarse purée is formed. Fold the purée back into the bean mixture. Add the cheddar cheese and cilantro, combine well. Mixture should resemble a coarse paste and be stiff enough to hold up in a scoop or spoon.

3 With an ice cream scoop or spoon, form 3–4 ounce portions. Sprinkle a plate with cornmeal and place scooped black bean portions on plate. Lightly dust black bean mixture with cornmeal and press down gently, forming a patty.

4 Preheat oven to 375°F. Spray a large nonstick pan with vegetable oil. Brown patty cakes for 2 minutes on each side. If pan is ovenproof, transfer to oven and bake for 15 minutes or until heated through. Or transfer patty cakes to a cookie sheet pan and bake.

EXCHANGES/CHOICES 1 1/2 Starch | 1 Vegetable | 1/2 Fat

Calories 165 | Calories from Fat 25 | Total Fat 3.0 g | Saturated Fat 0.7 g | Trans Fat 0.0 g
Cholesterol 0 mg | Sodium 440 mg | Potassium 265 mg | Total Carbohydrate 28 g
Dietary Fiber 4 g | Sugars 3 g | Protein 6 g | Phosphorus 110 mg

couscous and feta cakes

 6 servings

 1 cake

You may use traditional semolina couscous or whole-wheat for this recipe. Make these on a warm summer day, sit on the patio, and taste the flavors of the Mediterranean. Serve with your favorite marinara sauce over sautéed greens.

1 cup couscous, uncooked

1 tablespoon olive oil

1 cup red pepper, chopped

1/2 cup green pepper, chopped

1 cup red onion, chopped

2 cloves garlic, minced

2 tablespoons parsley, minced

1 cup reduced-fat feta cheese, coarsely crumbled

1/2 teaspoon white pepper

vegetable cooking spray

1 Preheat oven to 400°F. Bring 2 1/2 cups water to a boil, add couscous, and simmer for 5 minutes. Remove from heat, cover, and allow to cool for 10 minutes.

2 Heat 1 tablespoon olive oil in a nonstick pan over medium heat, sauté bell peppers, onion, and garlic for 4–5 minutes until softened. In a large mixing bowl combine all the ingredients, including the cooked couscous. Mix ingredients well and with a spoon or ice cream scoop form into 4-ounce portions. Scoop onto a plate or cookie sheet pan. Place a piece of wax paper or foil on top of portions. Flatten with the back of your hand.

3 Heat a large nonstick pan over moderate heat. Spray with vegetable cooking oil. Brown each side of the cakes for 3 minutes until golden in color. Place cakes on a cookie sheet pan and bake for 15 minutes until heated through.

EXCHANGES/CHOICES 1 1/2 Starch | 1 Vegetable | 1 Fat

Calories 190 | Calories from Fat 45 | Total Fat 5.0 g | Saturated Fat 2.0 g | Trans Fat 0.0 g
Cholesterol 10 mg | Sodium 290 mg | Potassium 195 mg | Total Carbohydrate 28 g
Dietary Fiber 3 g | Sugars 3 g | Protein 9 g | Phosphorus 145 mg

cowboy style "meatloaf"

 8 servings

 1/8 of the loaf

Hearty and full flavored, the spiced-up mixture of oats and beans is satisfying and soulful. Makes a great sandwich on a kaiser roll with sautéed onions and spicy ketchup.

2 teaspoons olive oil

1 cup diced onion

1 cup diced celery

1/2 cup diced green pepper

1/2 cup diced red pepper

1 jalapeño, minced

2 cloves garlic, minced

1 teaspoon cumin, ground

2 cups kidney or pinto beans, drained well and mashed slightly with fork

1 pound cooked, coarsely mashed potatoes, peeled

1 cup rolled oats (not instant)

1/3 cup bottled low-sugar barbeque sauce

1 tablespoon Dijon-style mustard

1 teaspoon salt

1/4 cup cilantro, minced

1 cup low-fat cheddar or Jack cheese (Optional) (You may use preblended Mexican cheese blend as well.)

1 Heat oil in a nonstick sauté pan over medium heat. Sauté onion, celery, green and red peppers, jalapeño, garlic, and cumin for 3 minutes.

2 Add mashed beans, cooked potatoes, and all remaining ingredients.

3 Place in a loaf pan and score the surface with a knife. Bake in a 375°F oven for 30 minutes until browned on top and heated through. If desired, glaze surface of loaf with 1/4 cup of additional barbeque sauce 10 minutes before end of cooking process.

EXCHANGES/CHOICES 2 Starch | 1/2 Fat

Calories 180 | Calories from Fat 20 | Total Fat 2.5 g | Saturated Fat 0.3 g | Trans Fat 0.0 g
Cholesterol 0 mg | Sodium 535 mg | Potassium 560 mg | Total Carbohydrate 34 g
Dietary Fiber 6 g | Sugars 4 g | Protein 7 g | Phosphorus 145 mg

eggplant risotto cakes

 8 servings

 1 griddlecake

Serve these griddlecakes with your favorite marinara sauce over sautéed spinach or pasta. If you like things spicy, add 1/2 teaspoon of crushed red chili flakes.

2 cups jasmine rice, uncooked

3 cups water

2 eggplants, peeled and diced into 1/2-inch cubes (each eggplant about 1 2/3 pounds)

Vegetable cooking spray

1 teaspoon dried Italian herb mixture*

1 teaspoon kosher salt

2 teaspoons olive oil

1 cup onion, chopped

2 cloves garlic, minced

4 ounces sun-dried tomatoes, chopped (reconstituted)

2 tablespoons capers

1 1/2 cups loosely packed fresh basil leaves

1 cup unseasoned breadcrumbs

1 Rinse jasmine rice in cold water. Cover rice with water, bring to a boil, reduce heat, and simmer, covered, for 25 minutes or until very tender.

2 Preheat oven to 375°F. Place diced eggplant on a cookie sheet pan and spray with vegetable cooking oil. Sprinkle with dried Italian herb mixture and salt. Bake eggplant for 35–40 minutes or until tender.

3 Heat olive oil in a nonstick pan over medium heat and sauté onion and garlic for 3 minutes until softened.

4 In a large bowl, combine cooked rice, sautéed onions, baked eggplant, sun-dried tomatoes, capers, basil, and breadcrumbs. Mixture should hold together well. If necessary, add a sprinkling of breadcrumbs to bind mixture.

5 Cool mixture slightly and form into 4-ounce portions with an ice cream scoop. Place portions on a plate lined with parchment or wax paper. Place another sheet of parchment or wax paper over scooped mixture and flatten lightly, forming a patty cake.

6 Spray a nonstick pan lightly with vegetable cooking spray and sauté cakes over moderate heat for 2 minutes on each side until golden brown. Place browned cakes on cookie sheet pan and bake for 20 minutes until heated through in a 375°F oven.

EXCHANGES/CHOICES 3 1/2 Starch | 2 Vegetable

Calories 330 | Calories from Fat 25 | Total Fat 3.0 g | Saturated Fat 0.6 g | Trans Fat 0.0 g
Cholesterol 0 mg | Sodium 540 mg | Potassium 785 mg | Total Carbohydrate 69 g
Dietary Fiber 7 g | Sugars 11 g | Protein 9 g | Phosphorus 155 mg

spinach, rosemary, and garlic cakes

 5 servings

 1 cake

This all-time favorite recipe pleases everyone from kids to grownups. You may also use fresh steamed spinach, chard, or kale to equal roughly 20 ounces cooked, instead of frozen, spinach. These are really super burgers loaded with antioxidants and flavor.

1 tablespoon olive oil

1 1/2 cups chopped onion

2 cloves minced garlic

2 (10-ounce) boxes frozen spinach, defrosted*

2 teaspoons minced fresh rosemary (or 1 teaspoon dried)

1/4 teaspoon nutmeg

1 pound peeled all-purpose potatoes, quartered

2 egg whites

1 cup unseasoned breadcrumbs plus 1/2 cup for crust

1/2 cup freshly grated parmesan cheese

1/4 teaspoon kosher salt

Vegetable cooking spray

1 Preheat oven to 375°F.

2 In a large nonstick pan, heat olive oil over medium heat. Sauté onion and garlic for 2 minutes, until softened. Add spinach that has been drained extremely well. Continue to sauté for another minute. Add rosemary and nutmeg. Place in a large bowl to cool and reserve.

3 Boil potatoes in water for 20 minutes or until tender. Drain, cool, and shred with a grater or in a food processor.

4 Add all remaining ingredients to the reserved spinach and combine well. (Mixture should be thick and well bound.) If mixture appears a bit loose, add more breadcrumbs. Form mixture into 4-ounce portions using a spoon or ice cream scoop. Place on a plate lined with parchment or wax paper. Place a sheet of parchment or wax paper over top of the cakes and press down lightly, forming patties. Sprinkle both sides of the cakes with the remaining crumbs.

5 Spray a large nonstick pan with vegetable oil. Brown spinach cakes over medium heat for 2 minutes on each side, until golden. Transfer to a cookie sheet and bake in a 375°F oven for 20 minutes or until heated through.

6 Serve over linguini with marinara or with spicy red beans.

*To drain spinach; place defrosted spinach into a colander and firmly press to remove all excess liquid.

EXCHANGES/CHOICES 2 1/2 Starch | 1 Vegetable | 1 Lean Meat | 1/2 Fat

Calories 295 | Calories from Fat 65 | Total Fat 7.0 g | Saturated Fat 2.1 g | Trans Fat 0.0 g
Cholesterol 5 mg | Sodium 560 mg | Potassium 665 mg | Total Carbohydrate 47 g
Dietary Fiber 7 g | Sugars 5 g | Protein 14 g | Phosphorus 195 mg

twice-cooked **sweet potato croquettes**

 8 servings

 2 croquettes

This is a wonderful dish to make for family and friends during the holidays or any time of the year, for that matter. Most supermarkets carry wild rice blends, such as Lundberg Farms, which include several varieties of brown and wild rice that are delicious and aromatic.

3 pounds sweet potatoes, baked (6 depending on size)*

1 cup wild rice blend, uncooked

1 cup walnut pieces

1/2 cup craisins (sun-dried cranberries), or you may substitute raisins or equivalent amount of any dried fruit (no sulfites please!)

1 tablespoon reduced-sodium soy or tamari

1 tablespoon grated gingerroot

1 cup unseasoned breadcrumbs

Zest of 1 orange (you may substitute 1 teaspoon dried peel)

1 teaspoon white pepper

1/2 cup natural sesame seeds (a mixture of black and natural seeds looks great)

Vegetable cooking spray

1 Preheat oven to 375°F. Cook rice according to directions on package by placing in pot with water, bringing to a boil, and simmering covered for 35 minutes or until tender.

2 Peel roasted sweet potatoes and place in a large bowl. Toast walnuts on a cookie sheet pan in preheated oven for 10 minutes until golden. Add the walnuts and all the remaining ingredients except the sesame seeds in the bowl. Mash the potatoes and combine well. With a spoon or ice cream scoop divide mixture into 4-ounce portions. With moistened hands, form the potato mixture into pyramid-shaped croquettes. Sprinkle lightly with sesame seeds and place on a cookie sheet pan lined with foil or parchment paper.

3 Spray lightly with vegetable oil and bake for 30 minutes until golden brown on the outside and heated through.

 CHEF STEVE'S TIP:

* TO BAKE SWEET POTATOES: Preheat oven to 375°F. Wash potatoes well and place on a baking pan. Pierce with a small paring knife and bake, turning occasionally, for 40–50 minutes until tender when a knife is inserted. You can bake the potatoes up to three days before making recipe.

EXCHANGES/CHOICES 3 1/2 Starch | 1/2 Fruit | 2 1/2 Fat

Calories 420 | Calories from Fat 145 | Total Fat 16.0 g | Saturated Fat 1.8 g
Trans Fat 0.0 g | Cholesterol 0 mg | Sodium 220 mg | Potassium 850 mg
Total Carbohydrate 63 g | Dietary Fiber 9 g | Sugars 15 g | Protein 10 g
Phosphorus 290 mg

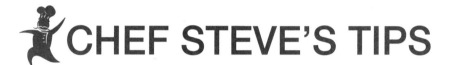# CHEF STEVE'S TIPS

brown rice vs. white rice

Brown rice is essentially the whole grain with just the inedible outer husk removed, which leaves vital nutrients and vitamins intact. Brown rice is higher in iron, manganese, and phosphorus than white rice. White rice has been polished and stripped of its husk, bran, and germ, which removes many of its essential elements. Generally brown rice takes longer to cook than white rice. Follow the package directions carefully when cooking either brown or white rice.

sticky brown rice cakes

 4 servings

 4 ounces

Short-grain brown rice or Arborio rice is essential to making these cakes bind together. The rice for these cakes can be cooked up to 2 days prior to forming burgers. Try these cakes with Picnic Salsa (page 129) or the Salsa Minestrone (131) over baked spaghetti squash.

2 cups short-grain brown rice (arborio rice may be substituted)

3 1/2 cups water

2 teaspoons sesame oil

2 tablespoons reduced-sodium tamari or soy sauce

1 tablespoon grated gingerroot

3 cloves minced garlic

1 cup grated carrot

1/2 cup pumpkin seeds

1 bunch scallions, minced

3 tablespoons cilantro, minced

Vegetable oil for spraying pan

1 Place rice, water, sesame oil, tamari, ginger, and garlic in a saucepot with a tight-fitting lid. Bring to a boil and lower to a simmer. Cook slowly for 35 minutes until rice is very soft and all the liquid is absorbed.

2 Add grated carrot, pumpkin seeds, scallions, and cilantro to the rice, cool slightly, and scoop into 4-ounce portions with an ice cream scoop or spoon. Form a patty shape and brown in a nonstick pan sprayed lightly with vegetable oil on both sides.

3 Bake for 10 minutes on a cookie sheet pan in a 375°F oven until heated through. Serve over sautéed spinach or with applesauce.

EXCHANGES/CHOICES 2 1/2 Starch | 1/2 Fat

Calories 220 | Calories from Fat 55 | Total Fat 6.0 g | Saturated Fat 1.0 g | Trans Fat 0.0 g
Cholesterol 0 mg | Sodium 195 mg | Potassium 280 mg | Total Carbohydrate 39 g
Dietary Fiber 4 g | Sugars 2g | Protein 6 g | Phosphorus 225 mg

udon noodle pancakes
with shiitake mushrooms

 8 servings

 2 pancakes

Crunchy on the outside and soft on the inside, these are amazing over a spinach salad served with Ginger Soy Drizzle (page 109). You may substitute an equal quantity of angel hair pasta, linguini, or spaghetti, if desired.

1 pound Udon noodles, uncooked

1 ounce dried shiitake mushrooms (3 ounces reconstituted)

1 cup carrots, shredded

1 bunch scallions, thinly sliced

1 cup water chestnuts, sliced

1 tablespoon gingerroot, minced

2 teaspoons garlic, minced

5 egg whites

3 tablespoons cornstarch

2 tablespoons reduced-sodium soy sauce or tamari

1 teaspoon black pepper, ground

1 1/2 cups breadcrumbs, unseasoned

Vegetable cooking spray

1 Preheat oven to 400°F.

2 Cook udon noodles in boiling water until very tender, drain well. Place cooked noodles and all the remaining ingredients in a large bowl. Mix gently, trying not to break up the noodles. Add more crumbs if mixture needs to be a little tighter in texture.

3 With a spoon or ice cream scoop, form mixture into 4-ounce portions and place on a plate or piece of wax paper.

4 Heat a large nonstick sauté pan over moderate heat. Spray with vegetable cooking oil and place noodle cakes into pan, being careful not to crowd them against one another. Brown each side for 3 minutes until golden in color. Place on a cookie sheet pan and bake for 15 minutes until heated through.

EXCHANGES/CHOICES 4 Starch | 1 Vegetable

Calories 350 | Calories from Fat 20 | Total Fat 2.0 g | Saturated Fat 0.4 g | Trans Fat 0.0 g
Cholesterol 0 mg | Sodium 340 mg | Potassium 310 mg | Total Carbohydrate 68 g
Dietary Fiber 5 g | Sugars 4 g | Protein 14 g | Phosphorus 145 mg

CHAPTER 4
Big Bowls, Plates, and Entrées

The definition of "meal" has changed significantly in the past decade. A meal used to be a plate with a piece of meat, a classic starch, and a vegetable. These were not always fresh and could be instant potatoes or frozen broccoli. I can still remember family grumblings if my mom made double vegetables and no starch. Those days are over. Even restaurants have changed their menu categories to reflect this new form of meal offerings. Big bowls are huge and entrées may mean a sampling of three small plates instead of one huge one.

These vegetarian recipes reflect new ideas for your meal planning. It could be a stew or soup loaded with intense, bold flavor and nutritionally rich ingredients, like **Trinidadian Curry Vegetables** (page 65) or a soulful **Autumn Skillet Paella** (page 74). Comforting and fulfilling doesn't mean complicated either. What could be better than a steaming bowl of fresh pasta with roasted garlic, tart lemon, and super-quality extra virgin olive oil? You may completely change your mind about tofu after you have prepared it pan-seared with herbs and a dollop of fiery salsa verde.

acorn squash stuffed with apple-almond-cranberry basmati pilaf

 4 servings

 1/2 stuffed acorn squash

Acorn squash are perfect carriers for this nutty aromatic basmati rice filling. You may roast the squash up to 2 days prior to filling each half with the stuffing to save valuable kitchen time. Unsweetened dried fruit may be found in most all-natural food grocery stores.

1 cup brown basmati rice

2 cups water

2 acorn squash (about 2 pounds each), halved and seeded

1 tablespoon olive oil

1 teaspoon butter

1 medium red or yellow onion, minced

1/3 cup chopped almonds

1/2 teaspoon minced garlic

1/2 teaspoon salt

1 apple, unpeeled, cored, and chopped

1/4 cup unsweetened dried fruit (look for raisins, cranberries, or cherries)

1 Combine the rice and water in a medium saucepan. Heat to a boil and cover. Reduce heat to simmer. Cook 40 minutes until tender.

2 Meanwhile, heat oven to 400°F. Place the squash, cut side down, on a greased, foil-lined baking pan. Roast 35–40 minutes until you can easily insert a fork from the skin side.

3 Meanwhile, heat olive oil in a small skillet over medium heat. Add butter and swirl until it melts. Add onions and cook 10 minutes, stirring often, until the onions become golden. Add the almonds and cook 5–8 minutes, stirring often, until the almonds give off an aroma. Stir in the garlic and salt. Cook 5 minutes. Remove pan from heat.

4 Add the onion mixture to the rice in the saucepan and toss to combine. Add the apple and unsweetened dried fruit and mix well.

5 Turn the squash halves over. Remove squash from the oven when done. Reduce heat to 300°F. Divide the rice mixture among the squash cavities, packing down the filling and mounding the top. (Leftover filling can be used as a side dish or refill component of the meal.) Cover the squash loosely with foil and return to oven. Bake 10 minutes.

EXCHANGES/CHOICES 4 1/2 Starch | 1/2 Fruit | 1 1/2 Fat

Calories 440 | Calories from Fat 100 | Total Fat 11.0 g | Saturated Fat 1.8 g
Trans Fat 0.0 g | Cholesterol 5 mg | Sodium 310 mg | Potassium 1365 mg
Total Carbohydrate 85 g | Dietary Fiber 17 g | Sugars 19 g | Protein 9 g
Phosphorus 295 mg

basil ginger cashew pilaf

 6 servings

 1 1/2 cups

Add any favorite vegetable to this rice, especially if you have trimmed and cut veggies lurking in your crisper. Feel free to add fresh minced scallions and sesame seeds to this dish as a garnish before serving.

2 cups white basmati rice

2 teaspoons peanut oil

2 teaspoons dark roasted sesame oil

1/2 medium onion, chopped

1 tablespoon fresh minced gingerroot

1 large carrot, peeled and chopped

2 stalks celery, chopped

1/2 red bell pepper, chopped

1/4 cup chopped cashews

1 tablespoon reduced-sodium soy sauce

1 cup fresh basil leaves, shredded

1. Cook the basmati rice according to directions, until just tender. Set aside. This step can be done up to 2 days prior to assembling recipe.

2. Heat peanut and sesame oils in a large nonstick sauté pan or wok.

3. Add onion, gingerroot, carrot, celery, pepper, and cashews. Sauté for 2 minutes until vegetables are barely tender and cashews start to pick up some color.

4. Add cooked rice and stir well. Sauté to heat through, adding a bit of water to encourage steaming of rice.

5. Add soy sauce and basil.

EXCHANGES/CHOICES 3 Starch | 1 Vegetable | 1/2 Fat

Calories 285 | Calories from Fat 55 | Total Fat 6.0 g | Saturated Fat 1.1 g | Trans Fat 0.0 g
Cholesterol 0 mg | Sodium 155 mg | Potassium 255 mg | Total Carbohydrate 51 g
Dietary Fiber 2 g | Sugars 2 g | Protein 6 g | Phosphorus 115 mg

claire's retro **stuffed peppers**

 6 servings

 1 pepper

This vegetarian version is from my mother, who would make them for a daily special. She owned a small mom and pop restaurant for many years. She was my culinary muse. Use your favorite marinara sauce for these peppers, which freeze well.

1 cup water

1/2 cup raw white basmati rice

1 tablespoon olive oil

1 medium onion, chopped

2 ribs celery, chopped

2 cloves garlic, minced

2 teaspoons dried leaf oregano

1/4 cup minced fresh parsley

10 ounces ground soy-based meat substitute (such as Gimme Lean or Boca)

Salt, to taste

Freshly ground black pepper, to taste

1 (24.5-ounce) jar low-sodium marinara sauce

1 (14.5-ounce) can no-salt-added diced tomatoes in juice

1 cup loose-packed basil leaves

6 medium red, yellow, or green bell peppers

1. In a small saucepan with a tight-fitting lid, bring water to a boil. Add basmati rice, stir, cover, and simmer 20 minutes until nearly tender. Transfer rice to a large mixing bowl.

2. Meanwhile, heat oil in a medium sauté pan or skillet and sauté onions, celery, garlic, and oregano 3 minutes until tender. Add sautéed vegetables to rice. Add parsley, soy beef, salt, and pepper to rice and mix to combine.

3. Combine marinara sauce, diced tomatoes, and basil leaves in a nonreactive medium bowl. Spoon 1 cup of tomato sauce mixture on bottom of a 2.5-liter baking dish.

4. Cut a 1/2-inch slice off top of each pepper. Remove seeds, reserving top pieces. Stuff peppers with rice mixture, leaving about 1/2 inch at the top empty. Place top of each pepper back in place and stand peppers in baking dish.

5. Pour remaining sauce over peppers. Cover loosely with foil and bake 50 minutes. Remove foil and bake an additional 15 minutes until lightly browned. Cool 10 minutes and serve.

EXCHANGES/CHOICES 1 1/2 Starch | 3 Vegetable | 1 Lean Meat | 1 Fat

Calories 265 | Calories from Fat 70 | Total Fat 8.0 g | Saturated Fat 1.0 g | Trans Fat 0.0 g
Cholesterol 0 mg | Sodium 555 mg | Potassium 1030 mg | Total Carbohydrate 40 g
Dietary Fiber 9 g | Sugars 12 g | Protein 16 g | Phosphorus 280 mg

enlightened tub of noodles

 6 servings

 1 1/2 cups

Think of this dish as a "kitchen sink" pasta dish for the whole family. It's quite forgiving as you can add any leftover diced vegetables and almost any pasta shape will work. It's also wonderful when served chilled. This is another of my mom's favorite dishes.

Salt, to taste

1 pound whole-wheat fettuccine or whole-wheat spaghetti, cooked al dente and drained

1 tablespoon extra virgin olive oil

1/2 cup chopped onions

3 cloves minced garlic

1/2 cup small broccoli florets

1/2 cup sliced snow peas

1/2 cup chopped zucchini

1/2 cup chopped red bell peppers

1/2 cup sliced mushrooms

1 teaspoon dried Italian herbs

1/4 cup freshly shredded Parmesan cheese

1. In a large pot of salted boiling water, cook the pasta according to package directions until al dente and drain.

2. Meanwhile, in a large nonstick skillet, heat the oil over medium-high heat. Add the onions, garlic, and broccoli and sauté 2–3 minutes. Add the snow peas, zucchini, peppers, mushrooms, and Italian herbs. Sauté the vegetables about 5 minutes until crisp but tender. Add the cooked pasta and combine well with the vegetables. Sprinkle with Parmesan cheese.

EXCHANGES/CHOICES 3 1/2 Starch | 1 Vegetable | 1/2 Fat

Calories 325 | Calories from Fat 35 | Total Fat 4.0 g | Saturated Fat 0.8 g | Trans Fat 0.0 g
Cholesterol 0 mg | Sodium 35 mg | Potassium 210 mg | Total Carbohydrate 58 g
Dietary Fiber 9 g | Sugars 3 g | Protein 14 g | Phosphorus 185 mg

pan-seared spicy asparagus with shiitake mushrooms

 4 servings

 1 1/2 cups

Serve this simple stir-fry over basmati or jasmine rice. If you love spicy flavors like I do, use a fresh Thai chili pepper or serrano chili, found in the produce section of many supermarkets or an Asian grocery store.

1 tablespoon canola oil

2 teaspoons Asian sesame oil

1 tablespoon minced gingerroot

2 cloves garlic, minced

1/2 teaspoon crushed red chili flakes

1 pound asparagus, bottom ends trimmed, cut diagonally into 1-inch lengths

1 (3.5-ounce) package shiitake mushrooms, stems removed and caps sliced thinly

2 teaspoons reduced-sodium soy sauce

1 tablespoon sesame seeds

1 Heat canola and sesame oils over medium heat in a large nonstick sauté pan or skillet. Add ginger, garlic, and chili flakes and sauté 1 minute.

2 Add asparagus and mushrooms: cook 4–5 minutes, stirring often, until asparagus are tender but al dente.

3 Add soy sauce and sesame seeds and combine well.

EXCHANGES/CHOICES 1 Vegetable | 1 1/2 Fat

Calories 90 | Calories from Fat 65 | Total Fat 7.0 g | Saturated Fat 0.8 g | Trans Fat 0.0 g
Cholesterol 0 mg | Sodium 100 mg | Potassium 170 mg | Total Carbohydrate 6 g
Dietary Fiber 2 g | Sugars 1 g | Protein 2 g | Phosphorus 55 mg

pasta pomodoro

 6 servings

 1 1/2 cups

Tomatoes are loaded with vitamin C and have been the subject of much research recently because they contain a phyto chemical called lycopene, which seems to be a powerful antioxidant or cancer-fighting agent.

3/4 pounds dried angel hair or linguine pasta

2 teaspoons extra-virgin olive oil

2 cloves garlic, peeled and minced

2 large tomatoes, chopped

1 cup fresh basil leaves, chopped

1 cup drained canned chickpeas

1/4 cup Asiago cheese, grated

1 tablespoon balsamic vinegar

1 teaspoon salt

1/2 teaspoon freshly ground black pepper

1 Cook the pasta according to package directions until al dente. Drain and set aside.

2 In a large nonstick skillet heat the olive oil over medium-high heat. Add garlic and tomatoes and sauté 2 minutes. Add basil, chickpeas, and cooked pasta.

3 Add cheese, vinegar, salt, and pepper. Combine well and heat through.

 CHEF STEVE'S TIP:

This simple dish enhances the natural flavor of the tomato by combining it with fresh basil and angel hair pasta for texture. If you like your pasta a bit spicy, add some dried red chili flakes or fresh minced jalapeño. I strongly recommend using an excellent quality extra virgin olive oil. Leftovers, if there are any, are great served chilled the next day. Serve this pasta dish with a great loaf of bread, field greens salad, and a good bottle of merlot or pinot noir.

EXCHANGES/CHOICES 3 Starch | 1 Lean Meat

Calories 280 | Calories from Fat 35 | Total Fat 4.0 g | Saturated Fat 1.0 g | Trans Fat 0.0 g
Cholesterol 5 mg | Sodium 465 mg | Potassium 305 mg | Total Carbohydrate 50 g
Dietary Fiber 5 g | Sugars 5 g | Protein 10 g | Phosphorus 155 mg

smoky chickpeas with spinach, eggplant, tomato, and manchego cheese

 4 servings

 1 1/2 cups

Discovered at an ancient tapas bar in Seville, I enjoyed this so much that one small plate was simply not enough. Smoked paprika was once obscure, but can now be found almost everywhere. You can serve this dish as-is or over rice, orzo, or couscous. Manchego cheese can be found in most cheese sections. You may use Parmesan if you can't find Manchego.

1 small eggplant, unpeeled and diced into 1-inch cubes

3 tablespoons extra virgin olive oil (divided use)

Salt, to taste

Pepper, to taste

1/2 Spanish onion, diced

1 clove garlic, minced

1 tablespoon smoked paprika

1 (15-ounce) can chickpeas, drained and rinsed

1 (14-ounce) can chopped, imported Italian tomatoes in juice

2 cups chopped fresh spinach or 1 cup frozen chopped spinach

1/3 cup crumbled Manchego cheese

1 Preheat oven to 375°F. Toss together eggplant, olive oil, salt, and pepper in large bowl. Spread on a baking sheet lined with foil or parchment paper and bake 30 minutes until golden brown and tender. This can be done up to 2 days prior to assembling recipe. Makes about 2 cups.

2 Heat oil in large nonstick sauté pan over medium heat. Add onion, garlic, and smoked paprika and sauté for 1 minute to soften onions. Add roasted eggplant chunks, chickpeas, tomatoes, and bring to a simmer. Cook for 5 minutes. Add the spinach and cheese.

EXCHANGES/CHOICES 1 Starch | 3 Vegetable | 3 Fat

Calories 290 | Calories from Fat 135 | Total Fat 15.0 g | Saturated Fat 2.9 g
Trans Fat 0.0 g | Cholesterol 5 mg | Sodium 310 mg | Potassium 650 mg
Total Carbohydrate 33 g | Dietary Fiber 9 g | Sugars 10 g | Protein 10 g
Phosphorus 195 mg

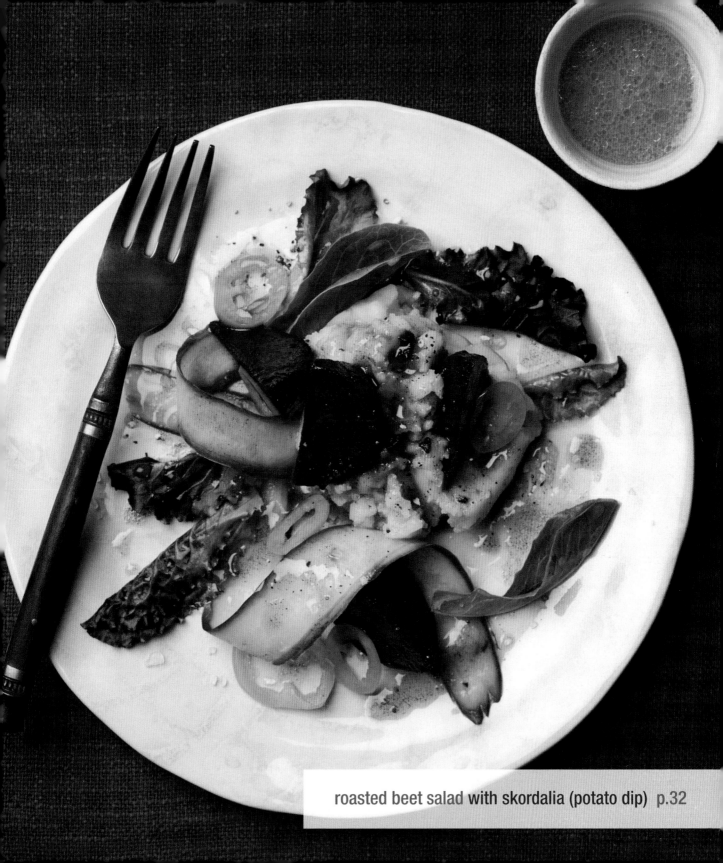

roasted beet salad with skordalia (potato dip) p.32

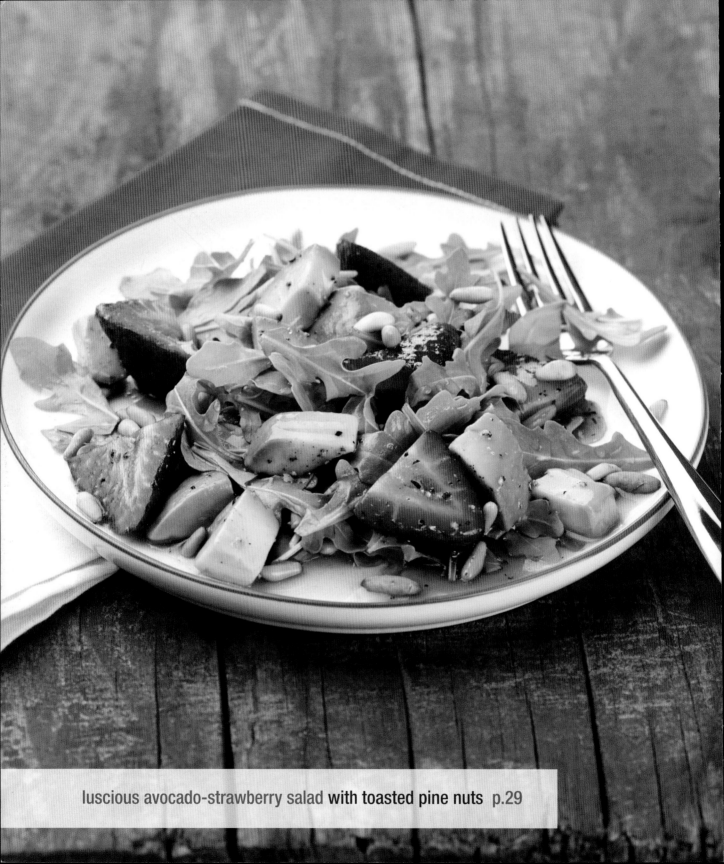

luscious avocado-strawberry salad with toasted pine nuts p.29

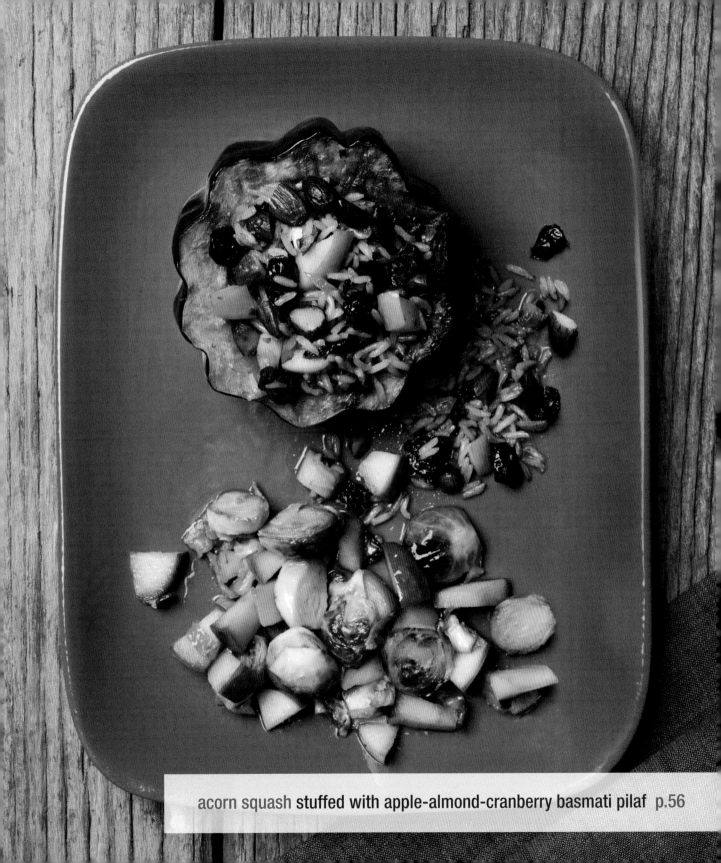

acorn squash **stuffed with apple-almond-cranberry basmati pilaf** p.56

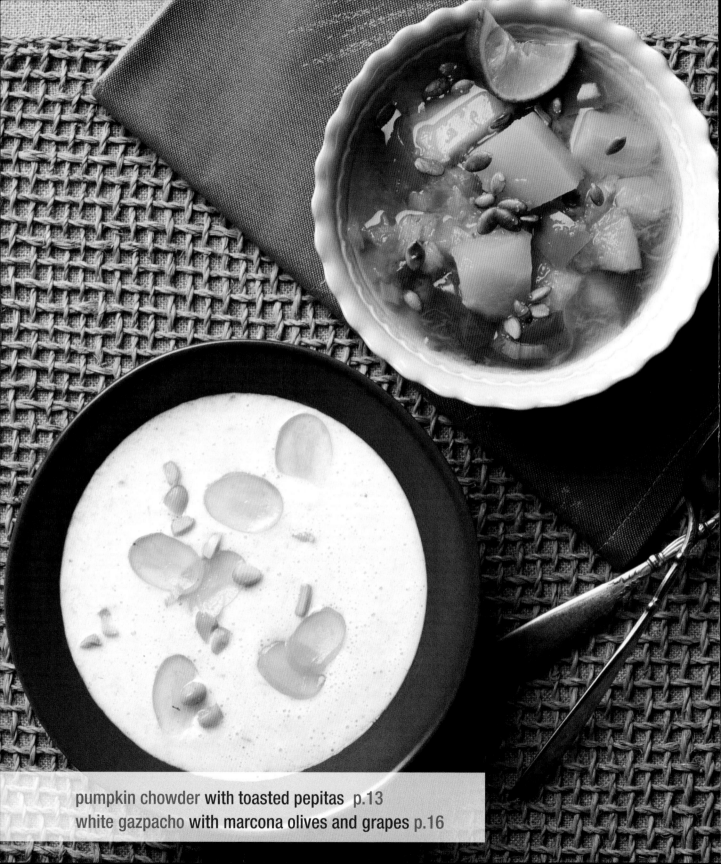

pumpkin chowder with toasted pepitas p.13
white gazpacho with marcona olives and grapes p.16

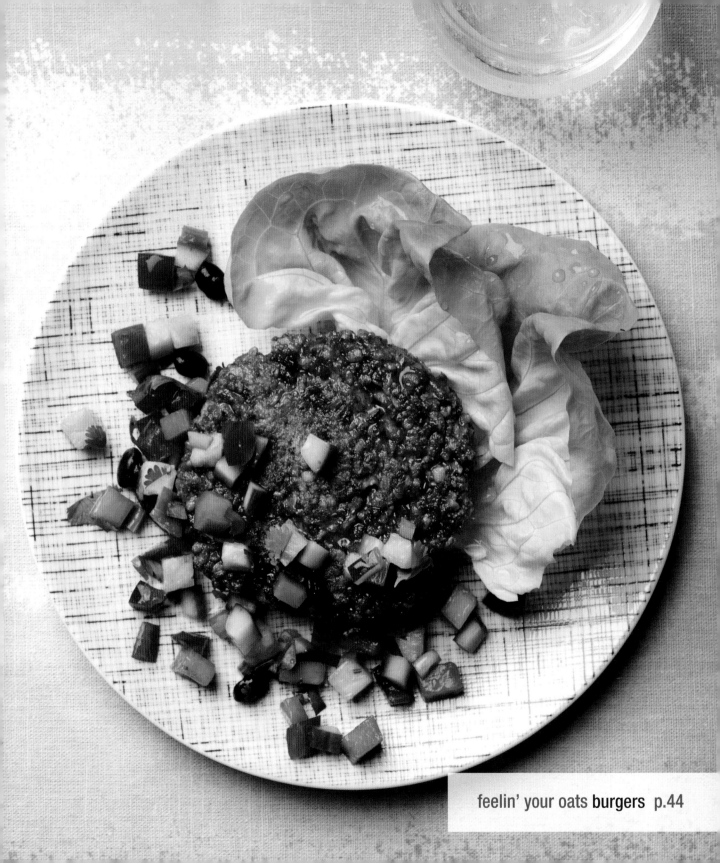

feelin' your oats burgers p.44

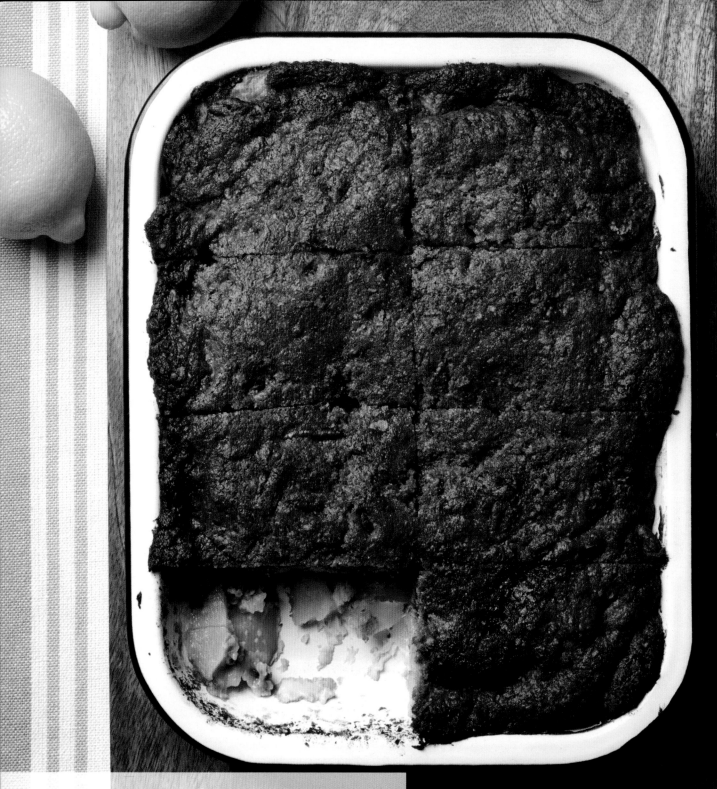

pear and stilton cobbler with pecans p.138

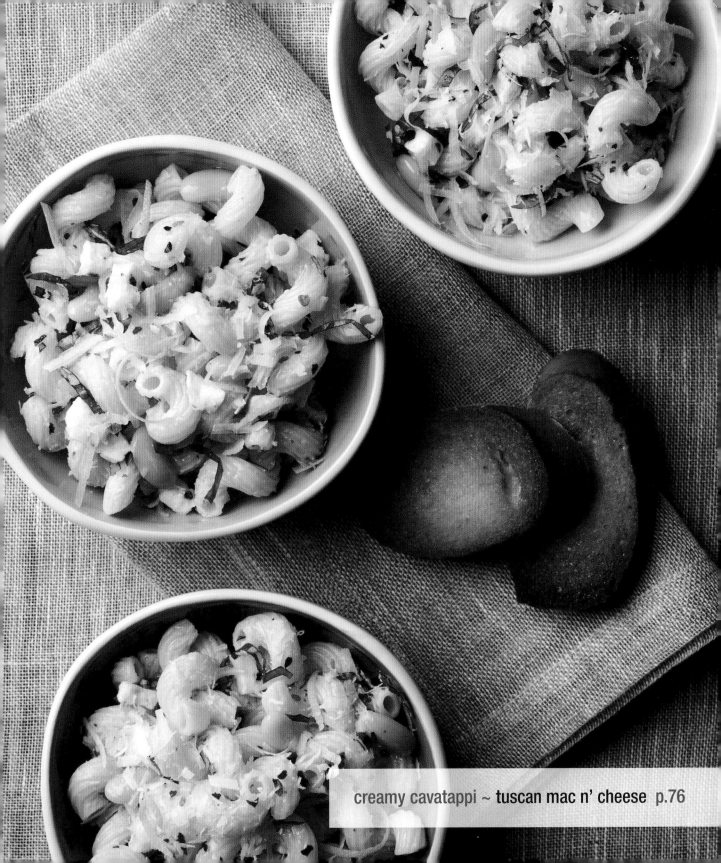

creamy cavatappi ~ tuscan mac n' cheese p.76

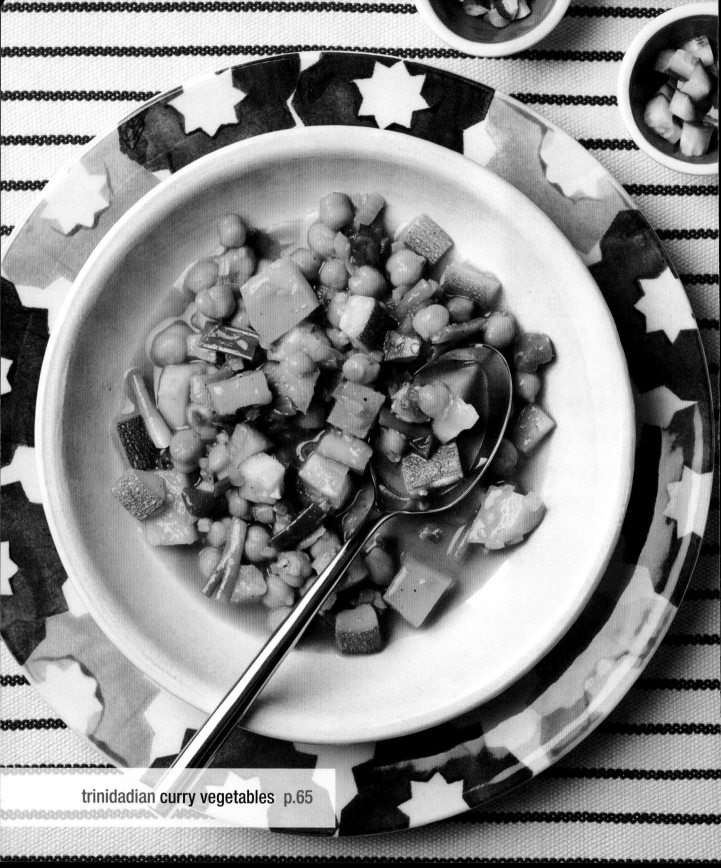

trinidadian curry vegetables p.65

zucchini, sweet pepper, and soy sausage pilaf

 6 servings

 1 1/2 cups

This one-pot meal is full of texture and bold flavors. The results of this dish are somewhere in between jambalaya and risotto. Tender zucchini and soy-based sausage form wonderful partners in this pilaf. If you like spicy, add some crushed red chili flakes.

1 tablespoon olive oil

1 small onion, chopped

1 medium red pepper, seeded and chopped

1/2 green pepper, seeded and chopped

1 stalk celery, chopped

1 (14-ounce) package Gimme Lean sausage

1/2 teaspoon dried thyme

1 1/2 cups white basmati rice

1 cup tomato, chopped (fresh or canned with juice)

1 3/4 cups low-sodium vegetable stock

2 medium zucchini, diced into 1/2-inch squares

1/2 cup frozen or fresh peas

Salt, to taste

Cayenne pepper, to taste

GARNISH

1 bunch scallions, minced

1 Heat oil in a large saucepot with a tight-fitting lid.

2 Sauté onion, peppers, celery, soy sausage, and thyme for 1 minute. Add rice and coat.

3 Add tomato and vegetable stock and bring to a boil. Lower to a simmer, cover tightly, and simmer for 25 minutes until liquid is absorbed and rice is almost tender.

4 Add zucchini, peas, and seasoning. Simmer for 2 minutes longer, covered. Allow to rest for 10 minutes before serving. Garnish with scallions.

 CHEF STEVE'S TIP:

Soy sausage is much better than it used to be and makes a great meat substitute in casseroles, stuffings, and sauces. There are several makers, with various flavors and spice profiles.

EXCHANGES/CHOICES 3 Starch | 1 Vegetable | 1 Lean Meat

Calories 300 | Calories from Fat 25 | Total Fat 3.0 g | Saturated Fat 0.5 g | Trans Fat 0.0 g
Cholesterol 0 mg | Sodium 435 mg | Potassium 1035 mg | Total Carbohydrate 53 g
Dietary Fiber 8 g | Sugars 7g | Protein 14 g | Phosphorus 230 mg

zucchini with rigatoni, pine nuts, and sun-dried tomatoes

 6 servings

 1 1/2 cups

In the U.S., zucchini hardly gets a chance to be the star ingredient. This recipe gives this beautiful and versatile squash a leading role as it soaks up any flavor that it is paired with. In this case, it works brilliantly with sweet, sun-dried tomatoes and crunchy pine nuts.

1 pound whole-wheat rigatoni pasta

1 tablespoon extra virgin olive oil

6 small zucchini, cut crosswise into 1/4-inch-thick rounds

3 cloves garlic, thinly sliced

1/4 cup rehydrated sun-dried tomatoes, chopped

1/4 cup pine nuts

1/3 cup low-fat ricotta cheese

1/4 cup freshly shredded Parmesan cheese

Salt, to taste

Freshly ground black pepper, to taste

1. Cook the pasta according to package directions until al dente. Drain, rinse in cool water, and set aside.

2. Heat the oil in a large nonstick skillet over high heat until oil is almost smoking. Add the zucchini slices, in one layer if possible, and allow to sit in the pan 2 minutes without disturbing them until they brown. Turn the slices and let sit 2 minutes without disturbing. Not disturbing the slices as they cook allows the natural sugars to brown and form a light crust with deep flavor.

3. Add garlic and sun-dried tomatoes, stirring well. Cook 1 minute. Add the pine nuts and cooked pasta. Toss to combine and heat 3 minutes before adding the cheeses, salt, and pepper. Toss to combine. Serve immediately.

 CHEF STEVE'S TIP:

To rehydrade sun-dried tomatoes, cover with boiling water and let sit about 20 minutes. Drain and chop.

EXCHANGES/CHOICES 3 1/2 Starch | 1 Vegetable | 2 Fat

Calories 390 | Calories from Fat 80 | Total Fat 9.0 g | Saturated Fat 1.5 g | Trans Fat 0.0 g
Cholesterol 5 mg | Sodium 125 mg | Potassium 510 mg | Total Carbohydrate 67 g
Dietary Fiber 10 g | Sugars 6 g | Protein 14 g | Phosphorus 260 mg

trinidadian curry vegetables

 4 servings

 1/4 recipe

Spicy, zesty, and full of intense palate-pleasing taste and aroma, this tropical stew will please everyone. Make a double batch and enjoy it all week.

1 tablespoon vegetable oil

1 onion, chopped

2 cloves garlic, minced

1 tablespoon gingerroot, freshly minced

1 medium zucchini, cut into 1/2-inch dice

1 jalapeño or serrano chili pepper, seeded and minced

1 medium all-purpose potato, peeled and cut into 1/2-inch dice

1 tablespoon good-quality curry powder

1 (15-ounce) can chickpeas, drained and rinsed

1 tomato, chopped

1/2 cup water or vegetable stock

6 scallions, chopped

Juice of 1 lemon

1 Heat oil over medium heat in a large saucepan. Sauté onion, garlic, and ginger for 2 minutes, stirring well.

2 Add zucchini, jalapeño pepper, and potato and sauté for 2 minutes longer. Add curry powder, chickpeas, tomato, water or vegetable stock, and scallions. Simmer for 20 minutes until potato is cooked through and a light sauce is formed.

3 Season with lemon juice and serve.

 CHEF STEVE'S TIP:

If jalapeños are too spicy for you, tone down the spice level by using a less spicy alternative of your choosing.

EXCHANGES/CHOICES 1 1/2 Starch | 2 Vegetable | 1 Fat

Calories 210 | Calories from Fat 55 | Total Fat 6.0 g | Saturated Fat 0.5 g | Trans Fat 0.0 g
Cholesterol 0 mg | Sodium 125 mg | Potassium 690 mg | Total Carbohydrate 35 g
Dietary Fiber 8 g | Sugars 8 g | Protein 8 g | Phosphorus 175 mg

steve's super three bean bowl

 10 servings

 1/10 recipe

Although this looks like a lot of ingredients, you simply place them in the pot and stir occasionally. You can top your chili with traditional garnishes, such as shredded cheddar cheese, low-fat sour cream or yogurt, chopped scallions, and chopped cilantro. If you have leftovers and you reheat this chili, you may need to add a little water because the beans and cracked wheat will absorb some of the liquid once it cools.

1 tablespoon extra virgin olive oil

1 medium onion, chopped

1 medium green bell pepper, cored, seeded, and chopped

1 medium red bell pepper, cored, seeded, and chopped

2 jalapeño peppers, seeded and minced

4 cloves garlic, minced

1 tablespoon chili powder

1 tablespoon dried leaf oregano

1 tablespoon smoked paprika

2 teaspoons ground cumin

1 (28-ounce) can diced tomatoes with juice

2 cups water, vegetable broth, or tomato juice

1/2 cup uncooked dried bulgur wheat

1 cup canned black beans, rinsed and drained

1 cup canned chickpeas, rinsed and drained

1 cup canned red kidney beans, rinsed and drained

1 to 2 tablespoons minced, canned chipotle chili in adobo

1 Heat oil in a nonreactive large pot over medium-high heat. Add the onions, peppers, garlic, chili powder, oregano, paprika, and cumin. Sauté 5–7 minutes until slightly softened and fragrant.

2 Add tomatoes and their juice; water, broth, or tomato juice; bulgur wheat; beans; and chili in adobo. Stir well.

3 Bring to a boil, reduce heat to a slow simmer, and cook, uncovered, 50–60 minutes, stirring occasionally, until the bulgur wheat is tender.

EXCHANGES/CHOICES 1 Starch | 2 Vegetable | 1/2 Fat

Calories 150 | Calories from Fat 20 | Total Fat 2.5 g | Saturated Fat 0.4 g | Trans Fat 0.0 g
Cholesterol 0 mg | Sodium 225 mg | Potassium 520 mg | Total Carbohydrate 27 g
Dietary Fiber 8 g | Sugars 6 g | Protein 7 g | Phosphorus 140 mg

loaded twice-baked potatoes

 4 servings

 1/4 recipe

Vegetarian bacon bits make a great addition to this dish. Any vegetable bits and pieces can be added to the filling. Keep in mind that hard vegetables need to be softened in a sauté pan or microwave before stuffing. The potato shells can be filled up to 2 days prior to baking.

2 large Idaho baking potatoes

1 cup chopped broccoli florets

1/2 cup chopped carrots

1/4 cup water

4 scallions, chopped

3 large mushrooms, chopped

1/2 cup plain, low-fat yogurt or light sour cream

Salt, to taste

Freshly ground black pepper, to taste

1/4 cup shredded low-fat cheddar, mozzarella, or Swiss cheese

Dash sweet paprika

1 Preheat oven to 375°F. Place potatoes on middle oven shelf and bake 40–45 minutes until tender. Remove and set aside to cool.

2 Place broccoli and carrots in a microwave-safe dish with water. Cover loosely with plastic wrap and microwave on high 2 minutes. Drain and rinse briefly in cold water, then drain and place in a small mixing bowl.

3 Add scallions, mushrooms, and yogurt or sour cream. Season with salt and pepper.

4 Cut each potato in half lengthwise and remove most of pulp with a teaspoon, leaving two shells to fill. Place white part of potato you scooped out of shells into bowl with other vegetables and mix lightly. Fill potato shells with mixture and sprinkle with cheese. Sprinkle with paprika. When ready to eat, place potatoes in a 375°F oven for 15 minutes until cheese is melted and potatoes are heated through.

EXCHANGES/CHOICES 2 Starch | 1 Vegetable

Calories 195 | Calories from Fat 20 | Total Fat 2.0 g | Saturated Fat 1.1 g | Trans Fat 0.0 g
Cholesterol 5 mg | Sodium 100 mg | Potassium 1075 mg | Total Carbohydrate 38 g
Dietary Fiber 5 g | Sugars 6 g | Protein 8 g | Phosphorus 215 mg

ravioli with arugula and hot chilies

 4 servings

 1/4 recipe

The success of this recipe depends on using good-quality ravioli. There are many varieties available with a variety of reduced-fat fillings and made with whole-wheat dough. Feel free to use spinach in place of arugula if you prefer.

1 pound uncooked, refrigerated, reduced-fat cheese ravioli of your choice

1 tablespoon extra virgin olive oil

1/4 teaspoon crushed dried red pepper flakes

Juice of 1/2 lemon

1 1/4 cup fresh arugula, washed with leaves intact

2 tablespoons freshly grated Parmesan cheese

Kosher salt, to taste

1 Cook ravioli according to package directions until al dente. This usually takes about 4 minutes.

2 Drain ravioli well and place in a large mixing bowl. Add remaining ingredients and toss until the arugula wilts slightly. Serve immediately.

EXCHANGES/CHOICES 2 Starch | 1 Lean Meat | 1 Fat

Calories 250 | Calories from Fat 65 | Total Fat 7.0 g | Saturated Fat 1.3 g | Trans Fat 0.0 g
Cholesterol 15 mg | Sodium 200 mg | Potassium 125 mg | Total Carbohydrate 36 g
Dietary Fiber 5 g | Sugars 2 g | Protein 11 g | Phosphorus 155 mg

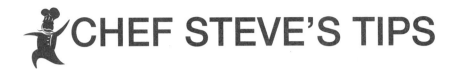

CHEF STEVE'S TIPS

alternative proteins

TOFU

Tofu, made from soybeans, is the most widely recognized vegetable protein source. Although tofu is available in silken or soft, firm and extra firm, the firmer it is the more it has the texture of meat. Use firm or extra firm for most dishes. Silken is used in dressings and desserts.

- You can marinate and grill the extra firm or firm varieties, make patties or croquettes, or even hollow it out and stuff it with grilled or sautéed vegetables.
- One trick to make tofu even more beef-like is to freeze a block of tofu overnight, then defrost and slice. It will be even firmer and steak-like in texture.
- Tofu is also available in a roasted, ground form. It is typically in the freezer section. Use it to make hearty chili or tacos.

TVP

- Textured vegetable protein is a concentrated soy product that can be used in place of ground beef for burgers, meat loafs, chilis, and stews. TVP also comes in chunks and packages that include all of the seasonings to make chili or stews.

TEMPEH

- Made from fermented soy and other grains, tempeh has a chewy texture and rich flavor and comes in various flavor varieties. It often contains other grains, such as quinoa, rice, or barley. Marinate it in your favorite barbeque sauce and grill it for a great alternative to beef burgers. I also use it in stews and chili.

sesame-seared tofu and edamame

 4 servings

 1/4 recipe

This dish offers a double dose of protein and even more flavor. Gomasio is a condiment made from toasted unhulled tan or black sesame seeds and salt that might also include bits of dried seaweed, chili peppers, lemon peel, and other spices. It is available in natural food markets and gourmet stores. You can substitute white sesame seeds, if you wish. Serve this over brown rice or quinoa.

1 tablespoon peanut oil

1 pound firm tofu, cut into 1-inch cubes

2 tablespoons sesame seeds or gomasio seasoning

1 cup frozen shelled edamame

1 tablespoon reduced-sodium soy sauce or tamari

8 scallions, cut into 1-inch lengths

1 Heat oil in a large nonstick sauté pan or wok over high heat. Toss the tofu with the sesame seeds or gomasio in a mixing bowl.

2 Add the tofu to the pan and sauté 2 minutes.

3 Add the edamame and continue to sauté 2 minutes.

4 Add the soy sauce and scallions and sauté until tender and the tofu is crisp.

EXCHANGES/CHOICES 1/2 Carbohydrate | 2 Lean Meat | 1 1/2 Fat

Calories 195 | Calories from Fat 110 | Total Fat 12.0 g | Saturated Fat 2.1 g
Trans Fat 0.0 g | Cholesterol 0 mg | Sodium 160 mg | Potassium 450 mg
Total Carbohydrate 9 g | Dietary Fiber 4 g | Sugars 2 g | Protein 15 g
Phosphorus 245 mg

spicy rigatoni
with lemon, chili, and spinach

 6 servings

 1/6 recipe

This is why classic Italian food is simple and brilliant. I made it even more nutritious by using a whole-wheat pasta and excellent-quality, extra virgin olive oil.

1 pound whole-wheat rigatoni or penne pasta

1 tablespoon extra virgin olive oil

3 cloves garlic, thinly sliced

1 teaspoon crushed red chili flakes

4 cups loosely packed baby spinach leaves

Juice of 1 lemon

1/2 cup shredded Parmesan cheese

1 Cook pasta al dente, according to directions. Rinse in cold water and drain well. This step can be done up to 2 days prior to preparing remainder of recipe.

2 Heat olive oil in a large nonstick pan over medium-high heat.

3 Add garlic and chili flakes. Sauté for 1 minute until garlic just begins to take on a golden color. Immediately add cooked pasta and sauté for 2 minutes to heat through.

4 Add spinach and sauté 1 minute longer until wilted. Add lemon juice and Parmesan.

EXCHANGES/CHOICES 4 Starch | 1/2 Fat

Calories 330 | Calories from Fat 40 | Total Fat 4.5 g | Saturated Fat 1.0 g | Trans Fat 0.0 g
Cholesterol 0 mg | Sodium 100 mg | Potassium 300 mg | Total Carbohydrate 62 g
Dietary Fiber 9 g | Sugars 3 g | Protein 12 g | Phosphorus 180 mg

chef's surprise package

 2 servings

 1/2 recipe

A number of these surprise packages can be made ahead and popped in the oven when you're hungry. They will keep well in the refrigerator up to 3 days prior to heating. You can add any fresh herbs or dried chili peppers to the packs as well. The aroma of the fresh herbs will envelope you and your guests upon opening the little packages.

1 cup cooked short-grain brown or brown basmati rice

2 (1/2-inch) slices firm tofu, cut lengthwise across a 1-pound block

4 large mushrooms, thinly sliced

4 thin slices Spanish or red onion

4 red bell pepper rings

1/2 cup shredded carrots

1 1/2 tablespoons reduced-sodium soy sauce or tamari

4 tablespoons shredded mozzarella cheese

1 teaspoon dried oregano

1 Preheat oven to 375°F. Place two 12-inch-long pieces of foil in front of you on work surface.

2 Place 1/2 of the rice in center of each piece of foil. Top each with 1 piece of tofu, then spread 1/2 of the vegetables over each piece of tofu in a neat pile.

3 Sprinkle each with 1/2 the soy sauce, cheese, and oregano. Bring edges of foil up around the filling and double-fold seam to seal or twist all edges together to resemble 2 big chocolate kisses. Place both packages on a baking pan and bake 30 minutes until heated through.

4 Carefully open each package to allow steam to escape.

EXCHANGES/CHOICES 1 1/2 Starch | 1 Vegetable | 1 Lean Meat | 1 Fat

Calories 230 | Calories from Fat 55 | Total Fat 6.0 g | Saturated Fat 2.2 g | Trans Fat 0.0 g | Cholesterol 10 mg | Sodium 530 mg | Potassium 465 mg | Total Carbohydrate 32 g | Dietary Fiber 4 g | Sugars 5 g | Protein 14 g | Phosphorus 290 mg

sautéed tempeh cutlets

 4 servings

 1 cutlet

Tempeh is a wonderful protein source for vegetarians. It's high in protein and fiber, but low in saturated fat. Tempeh comes in various flavors and takes on the taste of most ingredients it's paired with. It can be found in all natural food markets and many grocery stores.

2 sprays olive oil baking spray

1 teaspoon extra virgin olive oil

8 ounce packaged tempeh, cut into 4 equal "cutlets"

1 Spray skillet with olive oil spray, add oil, and heat over medium heat. Sauté cutlets 2–3 minutes per side until lightly browned outside and heated through. Top with Lemon Caper Sauce.

EXCHANGES/CHOICES 1/2 Carbohydrate | 1 Med-Fat Meat | 1/2 Fat

Calories 120 | Calories from Fat 65 | Total Fat 7.0 g | Saturated Fat 1.4 g | Trans Fat 0.0 g Cholesterol 0 mg | Sodium 5 mg | Potassium 235 mg | Total Carbohydrate 5 g Dietary Fiber 0 g | Sugars 10 g | Protein 10 g | Phosphorus 150 mg

LEMON CAPER SAUCE

1 tablespoon extra-virgin olive oil

1 shallot, minced

1 clove garlic, minced

2 tablespoons capers, drained

2 tablespoons minced parsley

Juice of 1 lemon

Freshly ground black pepper, to taste

1 In a small skillet or sauté pan, heat oil over medium heat. Add shallots and garlic and sauté 1 minute until softened. Add capers, parsley, lemon juice, and black pepper. Heat through and serve over Sautéed Tempeh Cutlets.

EXCHANGES/CHOICES 1 Fat

Calories 40 | Calories from Fat 30 | Total Fat 3.5 g Saturated Fat 0.5 g | Trans Fat 0.0 g | Cholesterol 0 mg Sodium 130 mg | Potassium 45 mg | Total Carbohydrate 2 g Dietary Fiber 0 g | Sugars 1 g | Protein 0 g | Phosphorus 5 mg

autumn skillet paella

 8 servings

 1/8 recipe

Plenty of vegetables from the garden and the pantry make this easy paella a hit for an impromptu gathering. Add a green or fruit salad and dinner is ready in a flash.

1 tablespoon olive oil

2 cloves minced garlic

2 cups chopped yellow onion

1 cup chopped celery

1/4 teaspoon saffron or turmeric

2 cups white basmati rice

3 cups (24 ounces) vegetable broth

1 cup canned, chopped, low-sodium tomatoes in juice

3/4 cup red bell pepper, seeded and cut into strips

3/4 cup green pepper, seeded and cut into strips

2 cups chopped kale or Swiss chard

1 cup chickpeas, drained and rinsed

1 cup frozen green peas

1 cup artichoke quarters, drained

1 tablespoon lemon juice

GARNISH

Lemon wedges

1 Heat oil in a large nonstick skillet with a tight-fitting lid over medium-high heat. Sauté garlic, onion, celery, and saffron (or turmeric) for 3 minutes until coated well. Add rice and continue to sauté for 1 minute longer.

2 Add stock, tomatoes, and peppers and bring to a boil. Lower to a simmer, cover tightly with lid, and simmer for 25 minutes until all the liquid is absorbed.

3 Fold kale, chickpeas, peas, and artichokes into rice. Recover and allow to rest for 10 minutes. Garnish with lemon.

EXCHANGES/CHOICES 2 1/2 Starch | 2 Vegetable | 1/2 Fat

Calories 275 | Calories from Fat 25 | Total Fat 3.0 g | Saturated Fat 0.5 g | Trans Fat 0.0 g
Cholesterol 0 mg | Sodium 505 mg | Potassium 610 mg | Total Carbohydrate 54 g
Dietary Fiber 6 g | Sugars 8 g | Protein 8 g | Phosphorus 180 mg

barely cooked tomatoes with basil and whole-grain pasta

 6 servings

 1/6 recipe

When summer tomatoes are at their peak, be sure to try this rustic pasta dish that is sure to please everyone at the table.

1 large garlic clove, smashed

1 1/2 to 2 pounds of ripe tomatoes, diced in 1/2 inch (Note: Tomatoes can be any combination or variety such as heirloom, cherry, grape, yellow, or other varieties.)

1 cup loosely packed whole basil leaves

3 tablespoons extra virgin olive oil

1/2 teaspoon crushed red chili flakes

1/2 teaspoon kosher or sea salt

1 pound whole-grain penne, fusilli, bowties, or rigatoni

Water to boil pasta

GARNISH

1/2 cup freshly grated Parmesan or Romano cheese

1 In a large mixing bowl, rub garlic vigorously around the surface of the inside. Leave small pieces of garlic that break in the bowl, then discard the main piece.

2 Add the tomatoes, hand tear the basil, and drizzle the olive oil over the mixture. Add the red chili flakes and salt. Allow to sit at room temperature while you cook pasta.

3 Cook the pasta al dente according to directions. Drain in a colander and add to the tomato mixture while pasta is hot. Serve with grated Parmesan or Romano cheese. Can be eaten hot or at room temperature.

EXCHANGES/CHOICES 3 1/2 Starch | 1 Vegetable | 2 Fat

Calories 390 | Calories from Fat 90 | Total Fat 10.0 g | Saturated Fat 2.1 g
Trans Fat 0.0 g | Cholesterol 5 mg | Sodium 275 mg | Potassium 355 mg
Total Carbohydrate 64 g | Dietary Fiber 10 g | Sugars 6 g | Protein 13 g
Phosphorus 205 mg

creamy cavatappi ~ tuscan mac n' cheese

 12 servings

 1/12 recipe

Cavatappi or corkscrew pasta captures the fresh shredded basil and creamy white beans in this Mediterranean version of a classic American favorite.

1 pound cavatappi pasta

3 1/2 tablespoons quality extra virgin olive oil

Juice of 1 fresh lemon

1 bunch basil, finely shredded

1/4 cup Parmesan-Reggiano cheese, shaved or micro-planed

1 (10-ounce) can cannellini beans with liquid

Salt and red chili flakes, to taste

1/2 cup fresh mozzarella, diced small

2 teaspoons finely shredded lemon zest

1 Cook pasta al dente, drain but DO NOT RINSE.

2 Place pasta back into the pot it was cooked in.

3 Add all remaining ingredients, adding the mozzarella last. Stir well to combine and top with lemon zest.

EXCHANGES/CHOICES 2 Starch | 1 Fat

Calories 215 | Calories from Fat 55 | Total Fat 6.0 g | Saturated Fat 1.5 g | Trans Fat 0.0 g
Cholesterol 5 mg | Sodium 50 mg | Potassium 140 mg | Total Carbohydrate 32 g
Dietary Fiber 2 g | Sugars 1 g | Protein 8 g | Phosphorus 105 mg

garden party roast vegetables **with pasta**

 6 servings

 1/6 recipe

Roast vegetables can be served in French bread, on focaccia, or tossed into pasta. Go ahead and get creative—use any seasonal vegetable or a favorite pasta shape like bowties or orrechiette (tiny disk-shaped pasta that look like little ears).

1 medium red pepper, large 1-inch dice

2 medium zucchini, sliced 1/2 inch thick

2 medium yellow squash, sliced 1/2 inch thick

1 small eggplant with peel, large 1-inch dice

1 red onion, peeled and cut into 1-inch-wide wedges

1/3 cup good-quality extra virgin olive oil

1/4 cup red wine or balsamic vinegar

Sea salt and ground pepper to taste

1 tomato, cut into wedges

1 bunch fresh basil, coarsely chopped (about 3 ounces)

1/2 cup pitted kalamata olives, chopped

Salt, to taste

1 pound dried spaghetti or shaped pasta, cooked according to package directions

1 Combine all ingredients except tomatoes, basil, olives, and pasta in a nonreactive container. Cover and marinate at least 1 hour at room temperature or overnight in the refrigerator.

2 Preheat oven to 450°F. Place all vegetables except tomatoes and basil in a nonreactive roasting pan. Roast 20 minutes or until almost tender, turning occasionally.

3 Add tomato wedges and roast 5 minutes longer. Add basil and olives and season with salt. Serve vegetables over or tossed into pasta.

EXCHANGES/CHOICES 3 1/2 Starch | 3 Vegetable | 3 Fat

Calories 505 | Calories from Fat 160 | Total Fat 18.0 g | Saturated Fat 2.3 g
Trans Fat 0.0 g | Cholesterol 0 mg | Sodium 195 mg | Potassium 720 mg
Total Carbohydrate 73 g | Dietary Fiber 8 g | Sugars 9 g | Protein 13 g
Phosphorus 195 mg

herb-crusted tofu
with fresh herb salsa verde

 4 servings

 1/4 recipe

Spoon the fresh Herb Salsa Verde over the tofu while the tofu is warm and it will soak up the flavors even more.

1/4 cup panko breadcrumbs

2 teaspoons Italian dried herb mix or oregano

1 tablespoon fresh minced parsley

1 teaspoon paprika or smoked paprika

1 pound extra firm tofu, cut into four, 1-inch thick steaks

1 tablespoon olive oil

FRESH HERB SALSA VERDE

2 tomatillos, chopped

2 scallions, minced

1/2 avocado, chopped

1/2 jalapeño, minced

1 teaspoon oregano, minced

1 teaspoon dill, minced

1 teaspoon cilantro, minced

1 tablespoon capers

Juice of 1/2 lime

1. In a small bowl combine panko crumbs, Italian dried herbs, parsley, and paprika.

2. Brush tofu with half the olive oil and press the tofu into the crumb mixture to coat it.

3. Preheat oven to 450°F. Place tofu steaks on a baking pan crust side up. Drizzle remaining olive oil over tofu. Cook for 8–10 minutes until brown.

4. In a medium bowl, combine the tomatillos, scallions, avocado, jalapeño, herbs, capers, and lime juice. Top tofu steaks with salsa and serve.

EXCHANGES/CHOICES 1/2 Carbohydrate | 2 Med-Fat Meat | 1/2 Fat

Calories 190 | Calories from Fat 115 | Total Fat 13.0 g | Saturated Fat 1.6 g
Trans Fa 0.0 g | Cholesterol 0 mg | Sodium 85 mg | Potassium 355 mg
Total Carbohydrate 10 g | Dietary Fiber 3 g | Sugars 2 g | Protein 13 g
Phosphorus 185 mg

sicilian stuffed mushrooms

 6 servings

 1/6 recipe

This recipe can become an entrée or appetizer by exchanging the small mushrooms for larger portobello mushrooms.

2 slices whole-grain bread, diced in 1/4-inch cubes

20–24 each baby portobello and crimini mushrooms (or 4 large portobellos)

1 tablespoon extra virgin olive oil

1/4 cup red onion, chopped

1/4 cup green pepper, chopped

2 cloves garlic, minced

1 teaspoon dried Italian herb spice mixture

1 egg white, beaten

1/4 cup low-fat or part-skim mozzarella cheese, shredded

2 tablespoons freshly shredded Parmesan cheese

1/4 cup roasted red peppers, chopped

1/4 cup artichoke hearts, chopped

1/4 cup fresh parsley, chopped

Juice of 1 lemon

1 Preheat oven to 375°F.

2 Place cubed bread on a baking pan and lightly toast in the center of the oven for 4–5 minutes until lightly browned. Remove from oven and set aside.

3 Remove stems from mushrooms and mince stems by hand or with a food processor. Set aside.

4 Heat oil in a large nonstick pan over medium heat. Add mushroom stems, onion, pepper, garlic, and Italian herbs and sauté for 5 minutes until softened.

5 Add bread cubes to sautéed vegetables. Add the egg white, cheeses, roasted red pepper, artichoke hearts, parsley, and lemon. Combine well.

6 Spoon the mixture into the mushroom caps. Place mushrooms on a baking pan on parchment paper and bake uncovered for 15–20 minutes until heated through and golden brown.

EXCHANGES/CHOICES 2 Vegetable | 1 Fat

Calories 100 | Calories from Fat 35 | Total Fat 4.0 g | Saturated Fat 1.0 g | Trans Fat 0.0 g
Cholesterol 5 mg | Sodium 150 mg | Potassium 530 mg | Total Carbohydrate 11 g
Dietary Fiber 2 g | Sugars 3 g | Protein 6 g | Phosphorus 170 mg

southwestern soy and potato bake verde

 8 servings

 1/8 recipe

I like making this dish the day prior to serving as it sets up like lasagna and can be sliced into squares. Even if you can't prepare it the day before, it's still delicious.

1 tablespoon olive oil

1 cup chopped Spanish onion

1 cup chopped green pepper

1 teaspoon ground cumin

1 teaspoon dried oregano

2 teaspoons smoked paprika, divided use

1 pound soy protein (such as Boca or Gimme Lean)

3 tablespoons tomato paste

4 cups chopped canned low-sodium tomatoes

1 cup low-sodium beef stock or water

3 minced chipotle chilies in adobo with 3 tablespoons of their juice

15-ounce can yellow hominy or corn, drained well

1 tablespoon lime juice

4 (3–4 ounces each) red skinned potatoes, unpeeled and sliced 1/4-inch thick in food processor or with mandolin

1 tablespoon olive oil

1/2 cup shredded low-fat cheddar or low-fat Monterey Jack cheese (optional)

1/2 cup chopped cilantro

1 Heat oil in a nonstick saucepan large enough to hold all ingredients. Sauté onion, green pepper, cumin, oregano, and 1 teaspoon of the smoked paprika for 4 minutes until vegetables are softened.

2 Add the ground soy protein and continue to sauté until vegetables are tender. Add the tomato paste, tomatoes, stock, chipotle chilies and their juice, hominy, and the lime juice. Simmer for 15 minutes until a smooth chili-like sauce is formed.

3 Line a 10 × 10 × 2-inch deep baking pan with half of the thinly sliced potatoes, overlapping them to cover the entire bottom. Pour the soy protein mixture over the potatoes and repeat the process with the remaining sliced potatoes to form an attractive overlapping pattern over the top.

4 Pat the potatoes down, drizzle with the olive oil, add the remaining smoked paprika, and place uncovered in the center of the oven. Bake 45 minutes until potatoes are tender and golden brown.

5 If using the shredded cheese option, scatter the cheese over the surface the last 5 minutes of baking. Garnish with chopped cilantro.

EXCHANGES/CHOICES 1 Starch | 2 Vegetable | 1 Lean Meat | 1/2 Fat

Calories 195 | Calories from Fat 45 | Total Fat 5.0 g | Saturated Fat 0.7 g | Trans Fat 0.0 g
Cholesterol 0 mg | Sodium 460 mg | Potassium 700 mg | Total Carbohydrate 28 g
Dietary Fiber 7 g | Sugars 7 g | Protein 16 g | Phosphorus 280 mg

grilled tofu (or tempeh) with avocado chili salsa

 4 servings

 1/4 recipe

Avocado Chili Salsa (page 82) can be served over grilled squares or slabs of tempeh, or extra-firm tofu. It's also fabulous over grilled eggplant or portabello mushrooms.

1 pound of either tofu or extra-firm tempeh, cut into 1-inch squares or in 1/2-inch slabs

MARINADE FOR THE TEMPEH (OR TOFU)

1 tablespoon corn, olive, or canola oil

Juice of 1 lime

1 tablespoon cilantro, minced

1 tablespoon reduced-sodium soy sauce or tamari

1 Combine all ingredients for the marinade. Place cut tempeh or tofu in marinade for at least 20 minutes or overnight in refrigerator.

2 Lightly spray a grill tray (one with holes) with a high-heat oil spray. Place tempeh or tofu in a single layer on the grill tray. Grill tempeh or tofu over a medium-high gas or charcoal grill for 3–4 minutes on each side. Remove from grill. Serve with Avocado Chili Salsa (page 82).

EXCHANGES/CHOICES 2 Vegetable | 1 Med-Fat Meat | 2 Fat

Calories 220 | Calories from Fat 145 | Total Fat 16.0 g | Saturated Fat 1.9 g
Trans Fat 0.0 g | Cholesterol 0 mg | Sodium 155 mg | Potassium 505 mg
Total Carbohydrate 11 g | Dietary Fiber 4 g | Sugars 3 g | Protein 13 g
Phosphorus 200 mg

avocado chili salsa

 4 servings

 1/4 recipe

You may use any favorite tomato for this recipe including Roma or even heirloom varieties. Try using a combination of yellow and red tomatoes, which, when combined with the green avocado, makes a great visual presentation. How much heat you prefer will determine the kind of chili you use. Serrano chilis are hotter than jalapeño peppers. Remove the seeds for a version with less kick. Make sure you wear gloves when handling hot peppers; it will save you much heartache later!

1 ripe avocado, cut into 1/2-inch chunks

1 medium ripe tomato, cut into 1/4-inch chunks

1/4 cup minced red onion

1 jalapeño or serrano chili, seeds removed, minced

1/4 cup minced fresh cilantro leaves

1 lime, juiced

Kosher salt, to taste

1 Combine all ingredients in a large, nonreactive bowl and mix gently with a spoon. Serve over the grilled tempeh or tofu. You may prepare the salsa up to a few hours before serving and store at room temperature in a covered container.

 CHEF STEVE'S TIP:

Avocados are ancient and date back to 10,000 B.C. They contain a much higher concentration of fats than most other fruits, which is mostly monounsaturated fat. They are truly a vegetarian delight.

EXCHANGES/CHOICES 2 Vegetable | 1 Fat

Calories 80 | Calories from Fat 55 | Total Fat 6.0 g | Saturated Fat 0.8 g | Trans Fat 0.0 g
Cholesterol 0 mg | Sodium 10 mg | Potassium 340 mg | Total Carbohydrate 8 g
Dietary Fiber 3 g | Sugars 2 g | Protein 1 g | Phosphorus 40 mg

pan-seared tofu
with garlic, lime & watercress

 4 servings

 1/4 recipe

This recipe will spark every taste bud! It's the ultimate combination of sweet, sour, and spicy, and the hint of soy sauce and lime juice makes the tofu sing with flavor.

1 tablespoon peanut or canola oil

1 teaspoon sesame oil

2 cloves minced garlic

1 tablespoon minced fresh ginger root

1 teaspoon chili paste or 1 minced fresh jalapeño chili

1 pound firm tofu, cut in 1-inch cubes

1/2 cup sliced red pepper

1 cup snow peas or sugar snap peas

1 tablespoon soy sauce or tamari

1 fresh lime, juiced

6 fresh basil leaves, shredded

1 cup watercress, heavy stems removed

1 Heat the oils in a large nonstick sauté pan or wok over high heat.

2 Add the garlic, ginger, and chili paste. Sauté for a few seconds and add the tofu. Cook the tofu for 2 minutes until lightly browned.

3 Add the bell pepper, snow peas, and continue to sauté for 2 minutes until vegetables are tender.

4 Add the remaining ingredients and serve immediately.

 CHEF STEVE'S TIP:

Serve with steamed rice or pasta and garnish with sesame seeds and thinly sliced scallions.

EXCHANGES/CHOICES 1/2 Carbohydrate | 1 Med-Fat Meat | 1 Fat

Calories 140 | Calories from Fat 80 | Total Fat 9.0 g | Saturated Fat 1.7 g | Trans Fat 0.0 g
Cholesterol 0 mg | Sodium 255 mg | Potassium 295 mg | Total Carbohydrate 6 g
Dietary Fiber 2 g | Sugars 2 g | Protein 10 g | Phosphorus 165 mg

mole marinara sauce

 4 servings

 1 cup

This mole marinara sauce is a quick version of the very complex Mexican mole sauce. Use this flavorful sauce over rice, pasta, or pour over baked tofu for a south of the border treat.

2 teaspoons olive or corn oil

1 cup red onion, minced

1 poblano or Anaheim chili, minced

1 teaspoon chili powder

1 teaspoon ground cumin

1 teaspoon dried oregano

1 (24.5-ounce) jar low-sodium marinara sauce

2 tablespoons unsweetened cocoa powder

1 tablespoon cilantro, minced

1 Heat oil in a large saucepan over medium-high heat. Sauté onion, chili, and spices for 2 minutes. Add the tomato sauce and simmer over low heat for 30 minutes.

2 Add cocoa powder and cilantro and serve.

 CHEF STEVE'S TIP:

Delicious on spaghetti squash, eggplant steaks, and grilled vegetables, I also love this sauce on French bread with melted Jack cheese.

EXCHANGES/CHOICES 1 Starch | 1 Vegetable | 1 1/2 Fat

Calories 175 | Calories from Fat 90 | Total Fat 10.0 g | Saturated Fat 1.3 g
Trans Fat 0.0 g | Cholesterol 0 mg | Sodium 445 mg | Potassium 745 mg
Total Carbohydrate 22 g | Dietary Fiber 5 g | Sugars 10 g | Protein 4 g
Phosphorus 105 mg

CHAPTER 5
On the Side

I can't tell you how many times I've been out to a restaurant with family or friends and it is the power of the side dish that makes my entrée decision. In fact, sometimes I opt for a collection of the side dishes listed on the menu. For me, the allure is variety. Sampling bold flavors that may have no apparent common thread at all. Like a food rebel, one can voluntarily buck the traditional menu categories and go wild tasting dishes from around the globe. That's exactly what lies inside this chapter. I bring the authentic flavor of **Athenian-Style Roast Zucchini** (page 86) to you directly from the little island of Chios, Greece, where a 94-year-old housewife made it for me in a wood-burning oven. The **Chickpea Pancakes** (page 92) are from the region of Liguria, Italy, and I still remember eating them scalding hot out of brown paper towels with a squeeze of lemon. Other sides in this chapter have become holiday traditions and have been passed down the generations for all to enjoy.

All of these side dishes are worthy of combining with one another to form a hearty main dish. Also if you wanted to "beef up" any of the side dish recipes, you can add any protein source like tofu, tempeh, seitan, or any "meat substitute" protein like Gardein for a more balanced dish.

athenian-style roast zucchini

 6 servings

 3/4 cup

This is a simple yet memorable dish with amazing flavor. That's what your company will say. I first tried this dish in a little sidewalk cafe in Athens.

8 small zucchini, cut in half lengthwise, then in 2-inch lengths

1 large ripe tomato, chopped

1 cup crumbled fat-free feta cheese

2 tablespoons extra-virgin olive oil

1 1/2 teaspoons dried oregano

Salt, to taste

Freshly ground black pepper, to taste

1 Preheat oven to 375°F.

2 Place zucchini in a 9 × 13-inch baking pan. Cover with tomatoes and feta cheese and drizzle with olive oil. Season with oregano, salt, and pepper.

3 Bake, uncovered, 25–30 minutes until zucchini is tender and golden brown.

EXCHANGES/CHOICES 1 Vegetable | 1 Lean Meat | 1/2 Fat

Calories 100 | Calories from Fat 45 | Total Fat 5.0 g | Saturated Fat 0.7 g | Trans Fat 0.0 g
Cholesterol 0 mg | Sodium 415 mg | Potassium 505 mg | Total Carbohydrate 9 g
Dietary Fiber 2 g | Sugars 5 g | Protein 8 g | Phosphorus 150 mg

cauliflower potato cheddar mash

 8 servings

 1 cup

These two vegetables make a perfect couple as creamy potatoes bond with the strong flavor of cauliflower. You can add broccoli as well for a delicious third wheel of taste.

1/2 large head cauliflower, separated into florets (about 2 cups)

2 pounds russet potatoes, peeled and cut into large chunks

Water

1/2 cup 2% milk, warmed

2 teaspoons butter, cut into small pieces

1/4 cup plain, fat-free Greek yogurt or sour cream

4 scallions, chopped

Kosher salt, to taste

Freshly ground black pepper, to taste

1/4 teaspoon fresh-ground nutmeg

1/4 cup shredded reduced-fat cheddar cheese

1 Place the cauliflower and potatoes in a large saucepan. Cover with water by about 1 inch.

2 Bring to a boil, reduce heat, and simmer 15–18 minutes until tender.

3 Drain well and return the cooked potatoes and cauliflower to the pan over low heat for 2 minutes to completely dry.

4 While smashing the vegetables with a potato masher or whisk, slowly add the milk, butter, yogurt, scallions, salt, pepper, nutmeg, and cheese. Mash until all ingredients are combined.

VARIATION
Spinach Mashed Potatoes: Instead of using the cauliflower, add 1/2 pound (8 ounces) frozen chopped leaf spinach to the potatoes the last 5 minutes of cooking. Drain well and proceed as directed above.

EXCHANGES/CHOICES 1 1/2 Starch

Calories 110 | Calories from Fat 20 | Total Fat 2.0 g | Saturated Fat 1.2 g | Trans Fat 0.1 g
Cholesterol 5 mg | Sodium 50 mg | Potassium 405 mg | Total Carbohydrate 20 g
Dietary Fiber 2 g | Sugars 2 g | Protein 4 g | Phosphorus 85 mg

festive vegetable gateau

 6 servings

 1 cup

This is one of the most elegant side dishes I know. It is a wonderful side dish but can also be served as an entrée over pasta, rice, or wilted spinach. Sweet caramelized onions complement the squash and tomatoes. Fresh thyme adds an herbal aromatic finish. The key to this dish is caramelizing the onions well and slicing the vegetables very thin. You may want to use a mandolin or Asian slicer. Also, use a good-quality extra virgin olive oil.

1 tablespoon plus 2 tablespoons extra virgin olive oil, divided use

2 large onions, chopped

Water, as needed

2 medium yellow squash, sliced very thin into rounds

2 medium zucchini, sliced very thin into rounds

2 medium tomatoes, sliced very thin into rounds

3 cloves garlic, sliced thin

4 sprigs fresh thyme, minced, or 1 teaspoon dried thyme

Salt, to taste

Freshly ground black pepper, to taste

1 Preheat the oven to 375°F. Heat 1 tablespoon oil in a large sauté pan or skillet over medium heat. Sauté the onions 12–15 minutes until very brown, adding a little water to the pan to prevent sticking, if needed. When the onions are well caramelized and very sweet, add about 1/4 cup water to the pan and scrape up any browned bits from the bottom of the pan with a wooden spoon.

2 Place onions with liquid from pan into a 2 1/2-quart casserole. Spread to form an even layer. Use the squash, zucchini, and tomatoes to form layers of vegetable over the onions. Form the rows by overlapping the vegetable rounds. Sprinkle the garlic and thyme over the vegetables. Drizzle with the remaining oil. Season with salt and pepper.

3 Bake uncovered 35 minutes until the vegetables are tender and lightly browned.

EXCHANGES/CHOICES 3 Vegetable | 1 Fat

Calories 120 | Calories from Fat 65 | Total Fat 7.0 g | Saturated Fat 1.0 g | Trans Fat 0.0 g
Cholesterol 0 mg | Sodium 15 mg | Potassium 560 mg | Total Carbohydrate 14 g
Dietary Fiber 3 g | Sugars 7 g | Protein 3 g | Phosphorus 85 mg

garlic spinach

 4 servings

 3/4 cup

The combination of caramelized garlic, wilted fresh spinach, and nutmeg is brilliant. If you have the time, purchase a jar of peeled garlic cloves. Bake them drizzled with olive oil in a 375ºF oven for 10 minutes until well browned. Use 1/2 cup of them in place of the sliced garlic. Use the remaining cloves on bread as a spread.

1 tablespoon olive oil

6 cloves garlic, thinly sliced

2 (10-ounce) bags prewashed spinach

Salt, to taste

Freshly ground black pepper, to taste

Pinch nutmeg

1 Heat oil in a large nonstick skillet over medium heat. Add garlic and sauté until lightly browned. Add spinach and stir well to combine.

2 Continue to sauté until spinach is wilted and bright green. Season with salt, pepper, and nutmeg.

EXCHANGES/CHOICES 1 Vegetable | 1 Fat

Calories 70 | Calories from Fat 35 | Total Fat 4.0 g | Saturated Fat 0.6 g | Trans Fat 0.0 g
Cholesterol 0 mg | Sodium 115 mg | Potassium 810 mg | Total Carbohydrate 7 g
Dietary Fiber 3 g | Sugars 1 g | Protein 4 g | Phosphorus 75 mg

new year's lucky round risotto

 6 servings

 1 cup

This dish is bound to bring luck because it's full of round ingredients such as arborio rice, beets, and onions. When cooked, the beets turn the rice an amazing ruby color as they sweeten the dish.

1 tablespoon olive oil

1 small red onion, chopped

2 cloves garlic, minced

2 medium beets, washed, peeled, and chopped

1 cup arborio rice

4 cups water or low-sodium vegetable broth

2 cups washed and shredded red chard, Swiss chard, spinach, or kale

1 tablespoon butter–canola oil blend (such as Land O' Lakes)

1/4 cup freshly shredded Parmesan cheese

Salt to taste

Freshly ground black pepper, to taste

1 Heat oil in a large saucepan over medium heat. Add onions, garlic, and beets. Sauté 4 minutes until vegetables are slightly softened.

2 Add rice and stir to coat well with oil. Add 1 cup broth at a time, stirring often and cooking slowly until each cup of liquid is absorbed before adding another cup.

3 Continue cooking 20 minutes. Add greens and continue to simmer 3 minutes. Add butter, cheese, salt, and pepper.

EXCHANGES/CHOICES 1 1/2 Starch | 1 Vegetable | 1/2 Fat

Calories 160 | Calories from Fat 45 | Total Fat 5.0 g | Saturated Fat 1.4 g | Trans Fat 0.0 g
Cholesterol 5 mg | Sodium 80 mg | Potassium 150 mg | Total Carbohydrate 26 g
Dietary Fiber 1 g | Sugars 2 g | Protein 4 g | Phosphorus 60 mg

the mother rice pilaf

 4 servings

 1/4 recipe

Rice pilaf is one of the world's great culinary gifts. It's not just a recipe, but the foundation for thousands of dishes from around the globe. It's a recipe that most home cooks don't know about because boxed rice pilaf mixes are preferred. But classic pilaf is such a simple dish to make, and it can be cooked from any rice or grain. This pilaf method can be made using one type of rice or grain or several types for a variety of textures and tastes.

1 tablespoon extra virgin olive oil, or butter

1/2 cup chopped Spanish onions

1 cup white jasmine or white basmati rice

1 1/2 cups low-sodium vegetable broth or water

2 bay leaves

Salt, to taste

Freshly ground black pepper, to taste

1 Heat the oil or butter in a small saucepan with a tight-fitting lid over medium-high heat.

2 Add onions and sauté 3 minutes until softened. Add the rice and continue to sauté until rice is coated well with oil or butter.

3 Add broth or water, bay leaves, salt, and pepper and bring to a simmer. Cover well, regulate heat so liquid simmers, and cook 25 minutes until all the liquid is absorbed and the rice is tender.

 CHEF STEVE'S TIP: RICE PILAF VARIATIONS

Add any of these ingredients during the last 5 minutes of cooking.
Tuscan Pilaf: Add 1/4 cup chopped fresh basil, 1 chopped medium tomato, 1 minced clove garlic, 1/4 cup grated Parmesan cheese.
Spanish Pilaf: Add 2 teaspoons paprika or smoked paprika, 1 chopped medium tomato, 1/2 cup drained chickpeas, minced jalapeño pepper, to taste.
Asian Rice Pilaf: Add 1 tablespoon low-sodium soy sauce, 1/4 cup frozen peas, 1/4 cup shredded carrots, 1/4 cup chopped red bell peppers, 1 scrambled egg.
Pumpkin Seed Pilaf: Add 1/4 cup shelled pumpkin seeds, 1/4 cup chopped cilantro, 1/4 cup queso blanco.
Nut and Fruit Pilaf: Add 1/4 cup nuts such as pecans, almonds, walnuts, pine nuts, pistachios, or macadamias and 1/4 cup dried fruit such as raisins, currants, chopped apricots, apples, or pineapple.

EXCHANGES/CHOICES 2 1/2 Starch | 1/2 Fat

Calories 210 | Calories from Fat 30 | Total Fat 3.5 g | Saturated Fat 0.6 g | Trans Fat 0.0 g
Cholesterol 0 mg | Sodium 55 mg | Potassium 135 mg | Total Carbohydrate 40 g
Dietary Fiber 1 g | Sugars 2 g | Protein 4 g | Phosphorus 90 mg

chickpea pancakes with cilantro

 8 servings

 3 pancakes

These unusual pancakes originated in Israel via Greece and are a family recipe, which my friend shared willingly. They are for a special occasion and can be served with fat-free Greek yogurt or a light drizzle of agave syrup. This recipe makes approximately 24 small pancakes.

2 teaspoons cumin seeds

2 teaspoons coriander seeds

1/2 teaspoon ground turmeric

6 to 8 slices fresh bread, preferably challah

1 (15-ounce) can chickpeas, drained and rinsed

6 whole eggs

1 tablespoon all-purpose flour

1 jalapeño pepper, seeded

1/2 cup fresh cilantro leaves, chopped

1 1/4 teaspoons kosher salt

1/2 teaspoon cayenne pepper

1/4 to 1/2 cup water

Canola oil spray, for sautéing

1 Heat a nonstick medium skillet over medium heat. Add the cumin seeds, coriander seeds, and turmeric. Shake the pan over the burner 2 minutes until the spices are lightly browned and very fragrant. Remove from heat and set aside.

2 In a food processer fitted with the metal blade, process the bread into crumbs. Set aside in a large mixing bowl.

3 Place the toasted spices, chickpeas, eggs, flour, jalapeño, cilantro, salt, and pepper in the food processor and process until the mixture is well combined and the texture of wet sand. Add to the breadcrumbs and mix to combine. Add enough water until mixture is consistency of thick pancake batter and will hold its shape on a spoon.

4 Spray a large nonstick skillet with the canola oil and place over high heat.

5 Place 2 tablespoons batter for each pancake into the hot pan, careful not to crowd them. Brown pancakes 2–3 minutes per side. Repeat until all batter is cooked.

EXCHANGES/CHOICES 1 Starch | 1 Lean Meat | 1/2 Fat

Calories 125 | Calories from Fat 45 | Total Fat 5.0 g | Saturated Fat 1.3 g | Trans Fat 0.0 g
Cholesterol 140 mg | Sodium 425 mg | Potassium 195 mg | Total Carbohydrate 12 g
Dietary Fiber 3 g | Sugars 2 g | Protein 8 g | Phosphorus 140 mg

cherry almond **couscous**

 9 servings

 1/9 recipe

This side dish is a memorable one that will bolster and complement a variety of main dishes. Cherries are loaded with antioxidants, fiber, and luscious flavor. When not in season, use unsweetened, pleasantly tart, jarred Morello cherries.

1 cup water

1 cup orange juice or sugar-free ginger ale

1 1/2 cups uncooked whole-wheat couscous

1 tablespoon extra virgin olive oil

1/2 cup pitted cherry halves, fresh or jarred (unsweetened)

1/4 cup dried cherries

1/4 cup sliced almonds

Juice of 1 lemon

Salt, to taste

Freshly ground black pepper, to taste

1/4 cup chopped fresh parsley

1 In a medium saucepan with a tight-fitting lid, bring the water and juice to a boil. Add the couscous and stir into the liquid. Turn off the heat, add the oil, cherries, almonds, lemon juice, salt, and pepper. Cover tightly and let sit on the burner 10 minutes.

2 Remove the cover, stir to fluff the couscous. Stir in the parsley. Serve warm or chilled the following day.

EXCHANGES/CHOICES 1 1/2 Starch | 1/2 Fruit | 1/2 Fat

Calories 165 | Calories from Fat 25 | Total Fat 3.0 g | Saturated Fat 0.4 g | Trans Fat 0.0 g
Cholesterol 0 mg | Sodium 5 mg | Potassium 165 mg | Total Carbohydrate 31 g
Dietary Fiber 3 g | Sugars 7 g | Protein 5 g | Phosphorus 90 mg

sweet potato and apple latkes

 5 servings

 4 latkes

Serve warm with applesauce, fat-free Greek yogurt, or both. These can be eaten for breakfast, as a dessert, side dish, or whenever…really! These are highly habit forming. This recipe makes approximately 20 latkes.

2 medium sweet potatoes, peeled and diced

Water

2 Granny Smith apples, peeled, cored, and grated

2 teaspoons lemon juice

2 tablespoons fat-free sour cream

1 egg, beaten

1/2 cup fresh breadcrumbs

1/3 cup chopped walnuts

1 teaspoon ground cinnamon

1/2 teaspoon ground cloves

Canola oil spray, for sautéing

1 Place potatoes in a saucepan with water to cover. Bring to a boil and cook 8 minutes until tender. Drain and mash in a bowl. Add the apples, lemon juice, sour cream, egg, breadcrumbs, walnuts, cinnamon, and cloves. Stir until smooth and thick. Mixture should hold together well on the end of a spoon.

2 Using a tablespoon or small ice cream scoop dipped in water, scoop up sweet potato mixture and place dollops on a large plate or pan sprayed lightly with oil. Flatten the mounds slightly.

3 Heat a large nonstick skillet sprayed with canola oil over medium-high heat. Add a few of the sweet potato latkes at a time, being careful not to crowd the pan.

4 Cook the latkes 3–4 minutes on one side until browned. Turn and brown on the second side. Repeat until all batter is cooked.

EXCHANGES/CHOICES 1 Starch | 1/2 Fruit | 1 Fat

Calories 150 | Calories from Fat 65 | Total Fat 7.0 g | Saturated Fat 0.9 g | Trans Fat 0.0 g
Cholesterol 40 mg | Sodium 60 mg | Potassium 235 mg | Total Carbohydrate 21 g
Dietary Fiber 3 g | Sugars 9 g | Protein 4 g | Phosphorus 80 mg

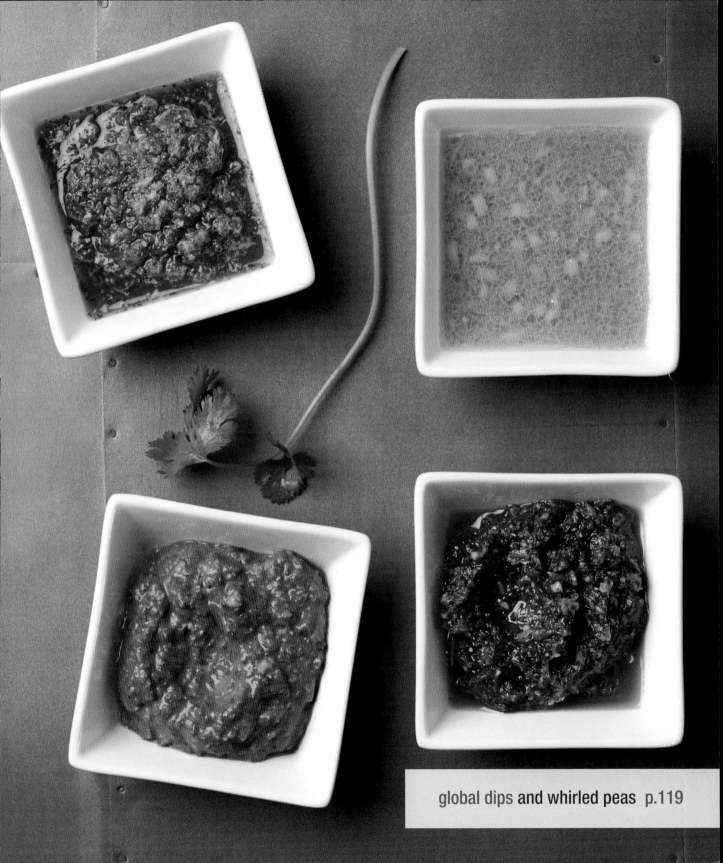

global dips and whirled peas p.119

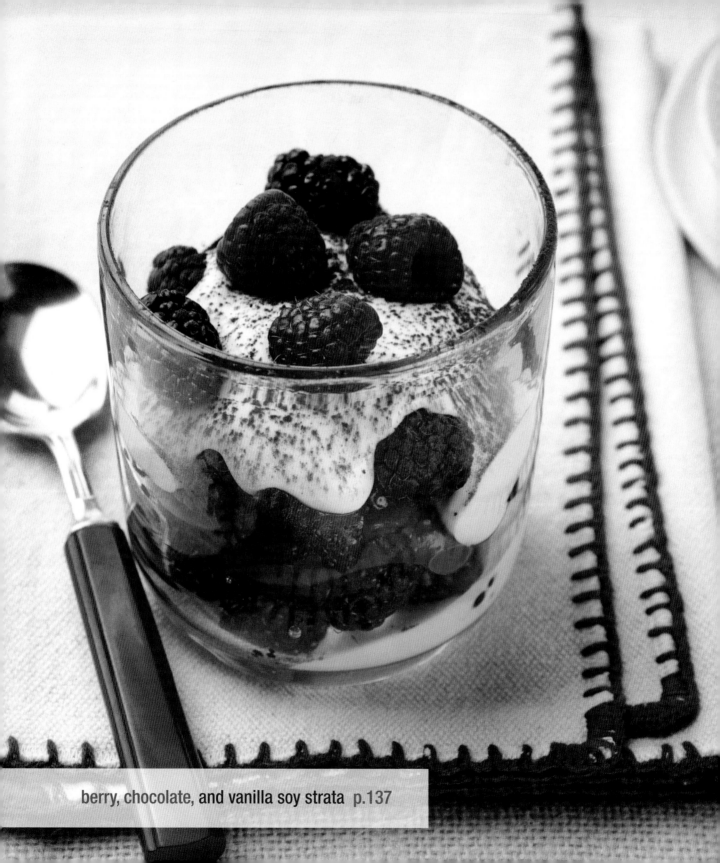
berry, chocolate, and vanilla soy strata p.137

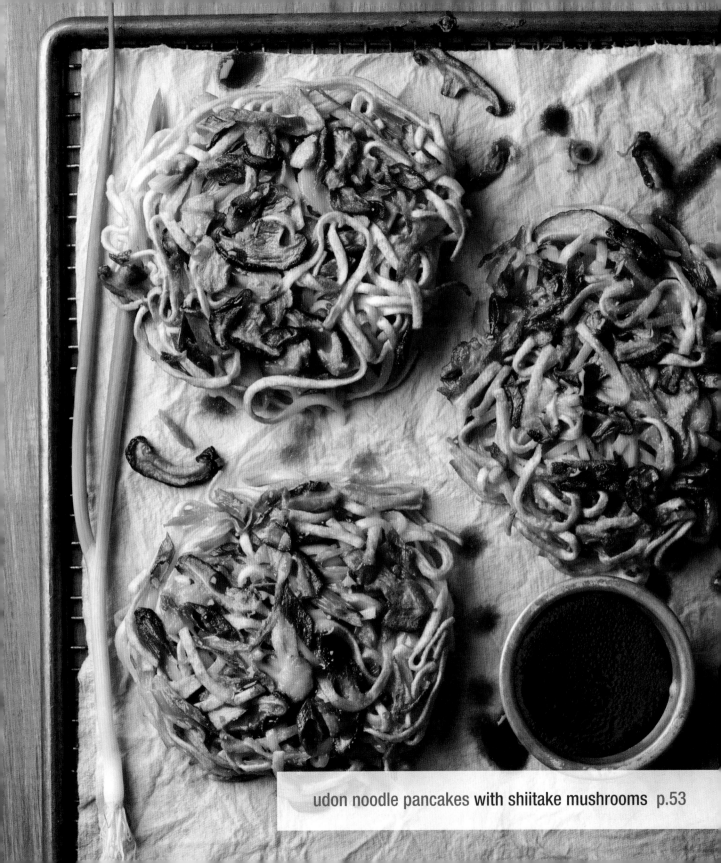

udon noodle pancakes **with shiitake mushrooms** p.53

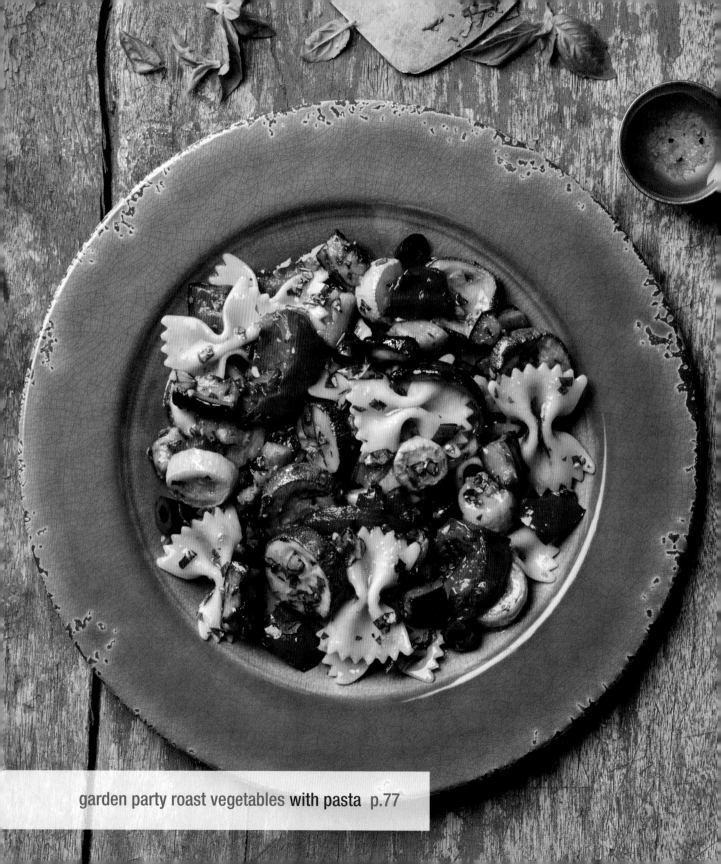

garden party roast vegetables with pasta p.77

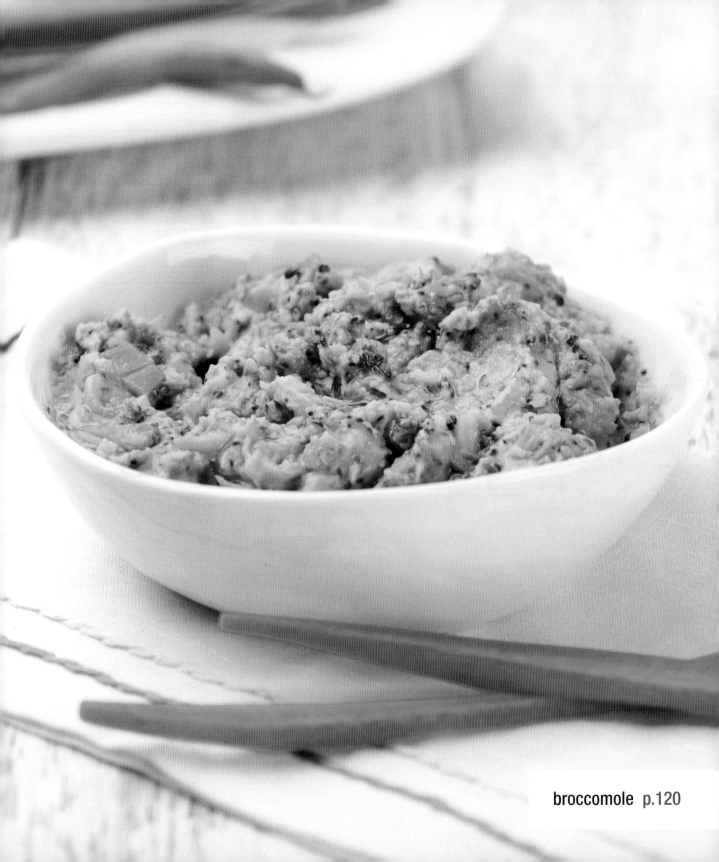

broccomole p.120

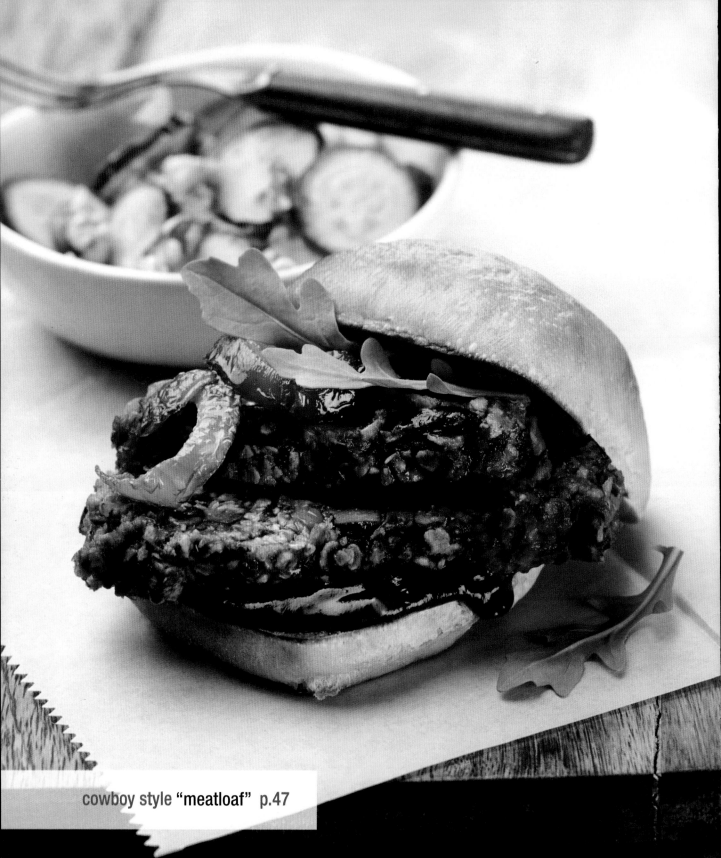

cowboy style "meatloaf" p.47

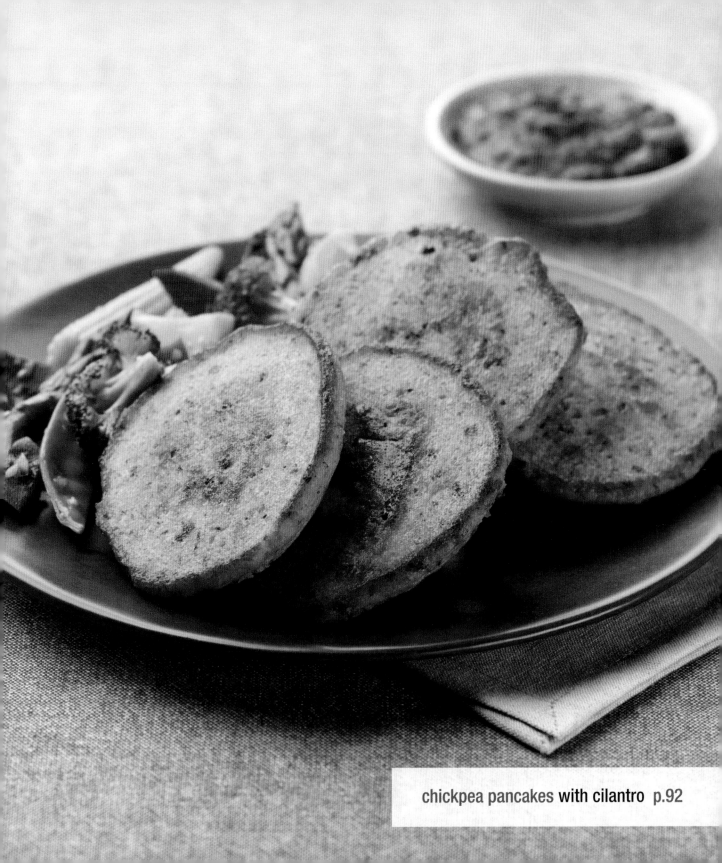

chickpea pancakes **with cilantro** p.92

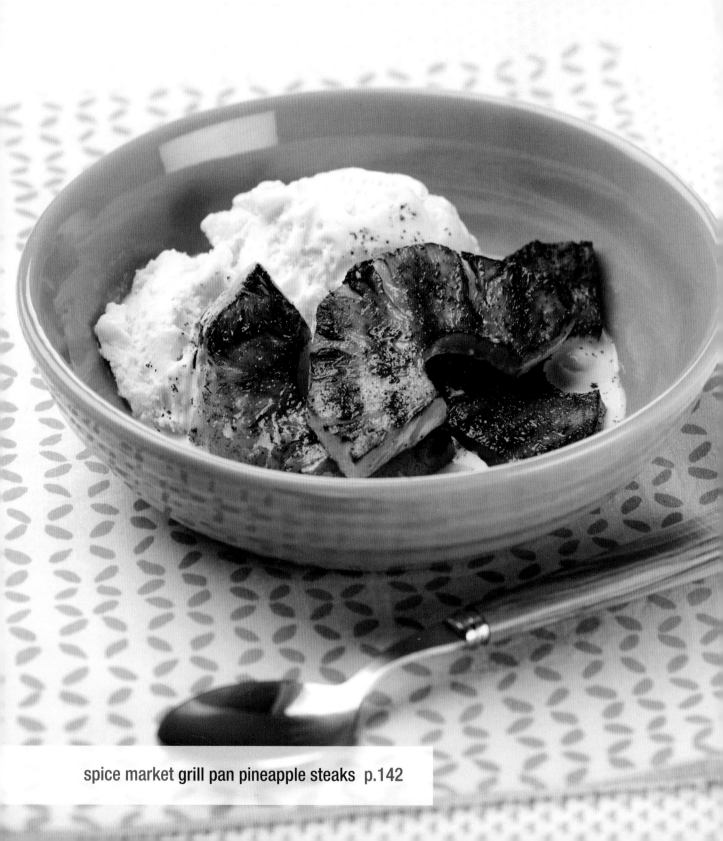

spice market grill pan pineapple steaks p.142

pan seared shredded brussels sprouts and apples

 8 servings

 1/8 recipe

My brother made this dish at Thanksgiving, and people loved it. Any firm, crisp apple will work in this recipe. Most people assume Brussels sprouts will be overcooked beyond recognition so this recipe is a welcome surprise. You can slice the Brussels sprouts in a food processor fitted with a 1/4-inch-thick slicing blade.

1 tablespoon olive oil

2 teaspoons unsalted butter

2 pints Brussels sprouts, bottoms trimmed and heads sliced 1/4-inch thick

2 apples, peeled, cored, and chopped (Granny Smith or gala apples recommended)

1 tablespoon honey

2 teaspoons lemon juice

Kosher salt, to taste

Freshly ground black pepper, to taste

1 Heat the oil and butter in a large nonstick skillet over medium-high heat until the butter begins to brown. Add the Brussels sprouts and apples.

2 Cook, stirring occasionally, over high heat 4–5 minutes until sprouts are just tender to the bite. Add the honey, lemon juice, salt, and pepper.

EXCHANGES/CHOICES 1/2 Fruit | 1 Vegetable | 1/2 Fat

Calories 65 | Calories from Fat 25 | Total Fat 3.0 g | Saturated Fat 0.9 g | Trans Fat 0.0 g
Cholesterol 5 mg | Sodium 10 mg | Potassium 205 mg | Total Carbohydrate 10 g
Dietary Fiber 2 g | Sugars 6 g | Protein 2 g | Phosphorus 35 mg

power applesauce

 8 servings

 1/8 recipe

I like to use honeycrisps for this recipe, but you can also use Granny Smith, Gala, Fuji apples, or any combination. Feel free to add antioxidant-rich fresh berries of any kind to the applesauce just when you turn the flame off, allowing the heat to gently wilt the berries and keep some of their character intact. Pomegranate molasses are available in Middle Eastern, Arab, and gourmet markets.

7 skin-on apples, cored and cut into 1-inch chunks

1 cup fresh or frozen cranberries

2 cinnamon sticks

1 (1-inch) piece gingerroot

1 cup pomegranate or cranberry juice

1/4 cup Splenda Brown Sugar Blend

1/4 cup pomegranate molasses

1. Place all ingredients in a nonreactive large heavy-bottom saucepan. Bring to a simmer over medium heat, cover, and cook 30–35 minutes until it forms a sauce. Stir occasionally so it doesn't burn on the bottom. Remove cinnamon stick and gingerroot chunk.

2. Mash fruit with a potato masher or, if you prefer a smoother sauce, place in a food processor fitted with the metal blade or a blender and purée.

EXCHANGES/CHOICES 2 Fruit | 1/2 Carbohydrate

Calories 140 | Calories from Fat 5 | Total Fat 0.5 g | Saturated Fat 0.0 g | Trans Fat 0.0 g
Cholesterol 0 mg | Sodium 0 mg | Potassium 370 mg | Total Carbohydrate 35 g
Dietary Fiber 4 g | Sugars 25 g | Protein 0 g | Phosphorus 20 mg

spring asparagus flashed in the pan

4 servings

1/4 recipe

While this recipe is wonderful over brown or basmati rice, feel free to use cooked orzo, quinoa, or even angel hair pasta. If you want to add protein, try diced tofu, seitan, or tempeh, added right after the asparagus hits the pan. I sometimes add crumbled ricotta salata cheese or queso blanco, a white cheese found in all supermarkets here in South Florida.

1 tablespoon olive oil

2 cloves minced garlic

1 pound fresh asparagus, sliced on the bias in 1-inch lengths

1/4 cup chopped sun-dried tomatoes

2 cups cooked brown or brown basmati rice

2 tablespoons minced tarragon or basil

2 teaspoons reduced-sodium tamari or soy sauce

1 Heat oil in a large nonstick pan or wok over high heat. Add garlic and asparagus, sauté for 3 minutes until slightly softened.

2 Add the sun-dried tomatoes, rice, tarragon, and tamari and combine well.

EXCHANGES/CHOICES 1 1/2 Starch | 1 Vegetable | 1/2 Fat

Calories 165 | Calories from Fat 40 | Total Fat 4.5 g | Saturated Fat 0.7 g | Trans Fat 0.0 g
Cholesterol 0 mg | Sodium 190 mg | Potassium 300 mg | Total Carbohydrate 27 g
Dietary Fiber 3 g | Sugars 2 g | Protein 5 g | Phosphorus 130 mg

roasted broccoli
with peppers and parmesan cheese

 4 servings

 1/4 recipe

Roasting broccoli at high heat in the oven brings out a rich flavor very different than just steaming or boiling it. Topped with a bit of Parmesan cheese, this dish takes your veggies to a whole new level.

1 head broccoli, ends cut 3–4 inches below the crown

1 red pepper, halved, seeded, and cut into strips

1 yellow pepper, halved, seeded, and cut into strips

1 red onion, cut into strips

2 cloves garlic, minced

2 tablespoons extra virgin olive oil

2 teaspoons Italian dried herbs

1/2 teaspoon kosher salt

1/4 cup shredded (not grated) Parmesan or Asiago cheese

1 Preheat oven to 475°F.

2 Place all ingredients except cheese in a large bowl and toss well to combine.

3 Spread vegetables out on a baking pan lined with parchment paper. Roast in center of the oven, turning occasionally, for approximately 25–30 minutes until broccoli is tender.

4 Sprinkle with Parmesan cheese.

EXCHANGES/CHOICES 3 Vegetable | 1 1/2 Fat

Calories 145 | Calories from Fat 70 | Total Fat 8.0 g | Saturated Fat 1.5 g | Trans Fat 0.0 g
Cholesterol 0 mg | Sodium 315 mg | Potassium 550 mg | Total Carbohydrate 16 g
Dietary Fiber 5 g | Sugars 6 g | Protein 5 g | Phosphorus 115 mg

grilled asparagus
with sun-dried tomatoes and parmesan

 4 servings

 1/4 recipe

Crisp jade green asparagus with the sweet flavor of sun-dried tomatoes and pungent Parmesan cheese create the perfect flavor trio.

1 pound asparagus, green, white, or a combination, stem ends trimmed

2 tablespoons extra virgin olive oil

1 tablespoon balsamic vinegar

1/8 teaspoon sea salt

1/8 teaspoon crushed red chili flakes

1/3 cup freshly grated Parmesan cheese

1/4 heaping cup sun-dried tomatoes chopped (not the oil-spacked variety)

1 Plunge asparagus spears into boiling water for 1–2 minutes depending on size. Drain and rinse in ice-cold water. This step can be done up to 2 days prior to serving asparagus.

2 Combine the olive oil, balsamic, salt, and red chili flakes in a small mixing bowl. Pour over the asparagus to marinate.

3 Heat a gas-fired or coal grill over medium-high heat and grill spears on a perforated grill pan for 4–6 minutes turning occasionally until golden brown.

4 Transfer asparagus to a serving platter, drizzle with leftover marinade, and sprinkle with parmesan cheese and sun-dried tomatoes.

EXCHANGES/CHOICES 1 Vegetable | 1 1/2 Fat

Calories 90 | Calories from Fat 65 | Total Fat 7.0 g | Saturated Fat 1.3 g | Trans Fat 0.0 g
Cholesterol 0 mg | Sodium 175 mg | Potassium 250 mg | Total Carbohydrate 5 g
Dietary Fiber 2 g | Sugars 3 g | Protein 3 g | Phosphorus 55 mg

coco rice with green onion

 8 servings

 1/8 recipe

Traditional Latin American rice is typically yellow in color. Here we use the natural spice turmeric for color and add a flavor twist by mixing in dried coconut and light unsweetened coconut milk. Dried, flaked, unsweetened coconut can be found in most Asian stores and natural food markets.

2 teaspoons canola or olive oil

1 cup chopped onion

1 1/2 cups white basmati rice

1/4 teaspoon turmeric powder

2 tablespoons flaked, dried coconut (unsweetened)

2 1/2 cups low-sodium canned or boxed vegetable broth

1/2 cup light unsweetened coconut milk

1/4 teaspoon kosher or sea salt

1/4 teaspoon freshly ground black pepper

1/2 cup chopped green onions (scallions)

1 Heat oil in a medium saucepan over medium-high heat. Add onion and sauté for 2 minutes until onions begin to soften, stirring constantly.

2 Add rice and turmeric powder and continue to sauté. Add coconut flakes and combine well.

3 Add broth and light coconut milk and bring to a boil. Immediately lower to a simmer, season with salt and pepper, cover with a lid, and simmer slowly for 20 minutes until rice is tender.

4 Uncover rice and allow to rest for 5 minutes. Mix lightly with a spoon to fluff rice. Fold in green onion and serve.

EXCHANGES/CHOICES 1 1/2 Starch | 1 Vegetable | 1/2 Fat

Calories 155 | Calories from Fat 25 | Total Fat 3.0 g | Saturated Fat 1.4 g | Trans Fat 0.0 g
Cholesterol 0 mg | Sodium 110 mg | Potassium 155 mg | Total Carbohydrate 29 g
Dietary Fiber 1 g | Sugars 2 g | Protein 3 g | Phosphorus 85 mg

fire-roasted tomato florentine

 4 servings

 1/4 recipe

Sometimes we overlook the beauty of simplicity. Fortunately, not in this dish made with garlic spinach nestled over juicy tomatoes. Romano and Parmesan cheese crown the tomato halves, adding a bit of crunch. Serve these as an appetizer, as a side dish, or over a bed of angel hair pasta drizzled with olive oil.

4 tomatoes, beefsteak, heirloom, or cluster

1 1/2 tablespoons extra virgin olive oil, divided use

1/2 cup chopped onion

3 cloves minced garlic

1 (10-ounce) package chopped spinach, defrosted (squeeze out excess moisture)

Pinch of nutmeg

Salt, to taste

Pepper, to taste

1/8 cup freshly grated Parmesan cheese

1 tablespoon grated Romano cheese

1/8 cup dried breadcrumbs, plain or seasoned

1 Cut the tomatoes in half and place them in a 9 × 9-inch baking dish, cut side up. Drizzle with 1 tablespoon olive oil

2 Heat 1 tablespoon of the oil in a sauté pan over medium heat. Add the onion and garlic and sauté for 1 minute. Add the spinach and sauté for 2 minutes longer. Season with nutmeg, salt, and pepper. Set aside.

3 Spoon some of the spinach mixture over each tomato until it is evenly distributed.

4 Combine the cheeses and breadcrumbs. Sprinkle it over the spinach-filled tomatoes and drizzle with the remaining olive oil.

5 Bake 15–20 minutes until the top is golden brown and the tomatoes are heated through.

EXCHANGES/CHOICES 3 Vegetable | 1 Fat

Calories 135 | Calories from Fat 65 | Total Fat 7.0 g | Saturated Fat 1.4 g | Trans Fat 0.0 g
Cholesterol 5 mg | Sodium 140 mg | Potassium 645 mg | Total Carbohydrate 15 g
Dietary Fiber 5 g | Sugars 6 g | Protein 6 g | Phosphorus 110 mg

pan roasted **harvest root vegetables**

 10 servings

 1/10 recipe

Roasting allows the sweet and delicate flavor of each root vegetable to shine through. Blanching the vegetables first in boiling water encourages natural vegetable sugar to caramelize over the surface and blend in with the subtle taste of thyme and lemon. As an option, try adding 2 pints of Brussels sprouts to the recipe.

3 cups red bliss potatoes, cut into small wedges (skin on)

2 cups carrots, peeled and cut into 1-inch-thick slices

1 1/2 cups parsnips, peeled and cut into 1-inch-thick slices

1 1/2 cups turnips, peeled and cut into small wedges

2 cups Spanish onion, peeled and cut into small wedges

1/3 cup extra virgin olive oil

1/8 cup minced fresh thyme (2 teaspoons dried)

5 cloves minced garlic

2 teaspoons fresh lemon peel (1 teaspoon dried lemon peel)

Juice of 1 lemon

Kosher salt, to taste

Freshly ground pepper, to taste

GARNISH

1 cup chopped fresh parsley

1 Preheat oven to 375°F.

2 Bring a large pot of water (10 quarts) to boil. Add the vegetables and simmer gently for 2 minutes. Drain and place in a large mixing bowl

3 In a small mixing bowl combine oil, thyme, garlic, lemon peel, and lemon juice. Mix the oil and spices into the reserved vegetables. Spread the vegetables out evenly on a baking pan, careful not to crowd them. Season with salt and pepper.

4 Roast uncovered, stirring occasionally, for 45 minutes until golden brown and tender. Sprinkle some water over the vegetables if they begin to stick to the pan

5 Garnish with the chopped parsley and serve.

EXCHANGES/CHOICES 1/2 Starch | 1 Vegetable | 1 1/2 Fat

Calories 135 | Calories from Fat 65 | Total Fat 7.0 g | Saturated Fat 1.0 g | Trans Fat 0.0 g
Cholesterol 0 mg | Sodium 30 mg | Potassium 425 mg | Total Carbohydrate 17 g
Dietary Fiber 3 g | Sugars 4 g | Protein 2 g | Phosphorus 65 mg

sesame seared pan veggies

 6 servings

 1/6 recipe

This is a colorful, all-purpose side dish that kids love as well as adults. Perfect over pasta, grains, or on a whole-wheat bun.

2 teaspoons peanut or canola oil

1 teaspoon dark-roasted sesame oil

1 large carrot, peeled and cut into coins

1 red pepper, cut into 1-inch strips, then diced on the diagonal to resemble diamond shapes

1 cup yellow squash, cut into half-moon shapes

1 cup small broccoli florets

1/2 cup baby corns, drained and rinsed well

1/2 cup sugar snap peas

1/2 cup asparagus spears, cut into 2-inch lengths

1 clove garlic, minced

2 teaspoons minced fresh gingerroot

2 1/2 ounces reduced-sodium soy or teriyaki sauce

1 tablespoon sesame seeds

1 Heat oils together over high heat in a wok or large sauté pan.

2 Add all vegetables, garlic, and ginger. Stir-fry, stirring constantly, for 3–5 minutes until vegetables are crisp tender.

3 Drizzle with soy sauce and add sesame seeds.

EXCHANGES/CHOICES 2 Vegetable | 1/2 Fat

Calories 70 | Calories from Fat 25 | Total Fat 3.0 g | Saturated Fat 0.5 g | Trans Fat 0.0 g | Cholesterol 0 mg | Sodium 455 mg | Potassium 270 mg | Total Carbohydrate 8 g | Dietary Fiber 2 g | Sugars 4 g | Protein 3 g | Phosphorus 65 mg

emerald sesame kale

 4 servings

 1/4 recipe

Simple and pure, this kale recipe can be eaten sautéed or raw as a salad if you prefer. I remember when no one ate kale, only the leaves were used as a garnish. Now, it is the darling of the vegetable kingdom. Make sure you remove the thick stem ends before slicing leaves.

1 tablespoon peanut or canola oil

2 teaspoons sesame oil, dark roast

2 cloves garlic, minced

1 tablespoon ginger root, minced

2 bunches of kale, either green or Lacinato (also called black or dinosaur kale), thinly sliced, washed well

1/2 teaspoon crushed red chili flakes

1 tablespoon reduced-sodium tamari or soy sauce

2 teaspoons sesame seeds

1 Heat oils together over medium-high heat in a large sauté pan or wok.

2 Add the garlic and ginger and sauté for 30 seconds until fragrant. Immediately add the kale with the moisture clinging to the leaves.

3 Sauté stirring constantly for 3–4 minutes until nearly tender. Add chili flakes, soy sauce, and sesame seeds.

EXCHANGES/CHOICES 2 Vegetable | 2 Fat

Calories 130 | Calories from Fat 80 | Total Fat 9.0 g | Saturated Fat 1.3 g | Trans Fat 0.0 g
Cholesterol 0 mg | Sodium 215 mg | Potassium 410 mg | Total Carbohydrate 11 g
Dietary Fiber 4 g | Sugars 2 g | Protein 4 g | Phosphorus 80 mg

smashed potatoes with kale and basil

 8 servings

 1/8 recipe

This is what happens when comfort food meets healthful food in a match made in dinner table heaven. This is a great side dish. If there are leftovers, they can be formed into a patty and browned in a sauté pan. I love this dish with eggs for breakfast as well.

2 pounds red bliss or Yukon gold potatoes

2 tablespoons extra virgin olive oil

4 cloves garlic, minced

1 bunch kale, heavy stems removed, chopped

1/2 cup low-fat milk, warmed

6 scallions, minced

1/4 cup fresh basil, chopped

1/2 cup Parmesan cheese, freshly grated

1/2 teaspoon black pepper, ground

1/4 teaspoon nutmeg, ground

1/2 teaspoons kosher salt

1/2 lemon, halved

1 Leave peels on potatoes, cut into chunks and boil in water, covered, until tender, about 15–18 minutes. Drain well and set aside in a large mixing bowl.

2 Heat olive oil and add garlic and kale. Sauté for 2 minutes and add mixture to potatoes in bowl.

3 Add all remaining ingredients to bowl except lemon and smash with a potato masher or large fork until combined but still chunky.

4 Squeeze lemon over potatoes and serve.

EXCHANGES/CHOICES 2 Starch | 1 Fat

Calories 190 | Calories from Fat 45 | Total Fat 5.0 g | Saturated Fat 1.4 g | Trans Fat 0.0 g
Cholesterol 5 mg | Sodium 220 mg | Potassium 660 mg | Total Carbohydrate 32 g
Dietary Fiber 4 g | Sugars 3 g | Protein 6 g | Phosphorus 180 mg

CHAPTER 6
Dress it Up:
Dressings, Sauces, and Marinades

After reading through and experimenting with the recipes in this chapter, you will understand that when you take a potato, a piece of bread, a slab of tofu, or even a wedge of iceberg lettuce and you dress it up with the right sauce, marinate it overnight, or rub it with a super spice blend, you can create a flavorful masterpiece that all will adore.

Many of the dressings, sauces, and marinades are interchangeable and can be used to drizzle over a fresh salad, marinate vegetables that will be chargrilled over a fire, or spooned over a black bean burger. This chapter is full of powerful flavor enhancers that you will want to keep in your refrigerator for weekly use. They allow you to prepare quick dinners in practically no time at all, when kitchen time is precious. Some of the recipes in this chapter will take your palate to places it has never been before. **Chimichurri sauce** (page 111), one of my all time favorites, has become a staple for me and I spread it on just about anything, including sandwiches. It's even popular in places I travel for work, especially Jamaica where it now vies with Jerk sauce for top billing. When I feel like comfort food, the **Pure Maple Glaze** (page 114) or **Creamy Buttermilk Dill dressing** (page 116) does the trick. Of course, I've been known to get in spicy moods, and the **Indonesian Sambal** (page 113) is the only thing that will do. Whatever the mood, breakfast, lunch, or dinner, we've got you covered.

bagna cauda

 16 servings

 1/16 recipe

This vegetarian version contains no anchovies, traditionally a part of this warm dip. Place the Bagna Cauda in a ceramic pot and place this pot in the center of a platter filled with washed and freshly cut carrots, zucchini, celery sticks, broccoli, or any other fresh vegetable that you like. You'll need approximately 6–8 cups of assorted fresh vegetables to serve 8 people.

3/4 cup extra virgin olive oil

5 cloves garlic, thinly sliced

6 basil leaves, minced

1 tablespoon fresh oregano, chopped

1/8 teaspoon crushed dried red chili flakes

Juice of 1/2 lemon

1 Heat oil in a small pot over medium heat without bringing it to a boil. Add remaining ingredients and heat 10 minutes. Pour into a ceramic pot.

CHEF STEVE'S TIP:

Bagna Cauda literally means "hot dip" and is eaten much like fondue. It typically contains anchovies and sometimes butter. It is typically eaten in fall and winter with carrots, fennel, peppers, artichokes, and cauliflower.

EXCHANGES/CHOICES 2 Fat

Calories 90 | Calories from Fat 90 | Total Fat 10.0 g | Saturated Fat 1.4 g | Trans Fat 0.0 g
Cholesterol 0 mg | Sodium 0 mg | Potassium 10 mg | Total Carbohydrate 1 g
Dietary Fiber 0 g | Sugars 0 g | Protein 0 g | Phosphorus 0 mg

ginger **soy drizzle**

 16 servings

 1 tablespoon

This simple Asian ginger vinaigrette can be used as a marinade or basting sauce for any vegetable or grilled tofu, as a dressing for salad, or as a dip.

1 tablespoon Dijon mustard

2 tablespoons grated peeled gingerroot

2 cloves garlic, minced

2 tablespoons canola oil

2 tablespoons dark-roasted sesame oil

2 tablespoons reduced-sodium soy sauce

1 tablespoon rice vinegar

Juice of 1/2 lemon

1 teaspoon honey

1/4 cup sugar-free ginger ale or water

1 Combine all ingredients well in a small mixing bowl. Store covered in the refrigerator for up to one week. Mix well before each use.

CHEF STEVE'S TIP:

Ginger is one of my favorite ingredients. It goes well with all Asian dishes. It can be pickled, made into tea, or baked into bread and cookies. In some countries, it is considered medicinal.

EXCHANGES/CHOICES 1 Fat

Calories 35 | Calories from Fat 30 | Total Fat 3.5 g | Saturated Fat 0.4 g | Trans Fat 0.0 g
Cholesterol 0 mg | Sodium 90 mg | Potassium 10 mg | Total Carbohydrate 1 g
Dietary Fiber 0 g | Sugars 1g | Protein 0 g | Phosphorus 0 mg

cucumber, pineapple, and papaya salsa

 16 servings

 2 1/2 tablespoons

Exotic, refreshing, and addictive are the three words that immediately come to mind when I think about this salsa. Great on everything, especially grilled entrées, or cooked rice, this salsa hits all the taste sensors at once.

1 cup seeded, peeled, and diced cucumbers (you can use English seedless cucumbers in place)

1 cup diced ripe pineapple

1/2 cup diced ripe papaya

1/4 cup minced red onions

1/2 cup diced ripe tomatoes

1 tablespoon lime juice

2 tablespoons minced cilantro

1/4 cup cooked black beans (optional)

2 teaspoons minced, seeded jalapeño

1 Combine all ingredients well in a nonreactive container and chill. Will keep refrigerated for 3–4 days.

EXCHANGES/CHOICES Free Food

Calories 10 | Calories from Fat 0 | Total Fat 0.0 g | Saturated Fat 0.0 g | Trans Fat 0.0 g
Cholesterol 0 mg | Sodium 0 mg | Potassium 55 mg | Total Carbohydrate 3 g
Dietary Fiber 0 g | Sugars 2 g | Protein 0 g | Phosphorus 5 mg

chimichurri **cilantro sauce**

 16 servings

 1 tablespoon

This sauce can be made with parsley, basil, or any favorite herb if you are not a cilantro fan. It's wonderful on grilled tofu, tempeh, or on grilled vegetables of every sort. Try it on a grilled vegetable sandwich on whole-grain bread.

2 cups packed cilantro leaves

1/2 cup packed flat-leaf parsley

3 cloves garlic

3 scallions

1/2 cup extra-virgin olive oil

1 jalapeño pepper, seeded and chopped

2 teaspoons kosher salt

Juice of 1 lime

1 Make sure cilantro and parsley are well washed. Place all ingredients in a blender or food processor fitted with metal blade and process 45 seconds or until combined well.

EXCHANGES/CHOICES 1 1/2 Fat

Calories 65 | Calories from Fat 65 | Total Fat 7.0 g | Saturated Fat 0.9 g | Trans Fat 0.0 g
Cholesterol 0 mg | Sodium 245 mg | Potassium 45 mg | Total Carbohydrate 1 g
Dietary Fiber 0 g | Sugars 0 g | Protein 0 g | Phosphorus 5 mg

chef steve's diablo dipping sauce

 16 servings

 1 tablespoon

I normally make this with canned chipotle chili peppers in adobo sauce. You can find these smoky, sweet, and spicy smoked jalapeños in the ethnic foods aisle of any supermarket. They are hot! Use this spicy dipping sauce on freshly cut vegetables or over steamed broccoli, green beans, or cauliflower.

2 chilies in adobo sauce (canned)

2 roasted red peppers (canned or jarred), drained

1 tablespoon tomato paste

1/4 cup almonds or walnuts

1/4 cup extra-virgin olive oil

2 tablespoons red wine vinegar

Salt, to taste

1   Place all ingredients in a blender or food processor fitted with metal blade and process or blend 45 seconds until combined well and smooth.

EXCHANGES/CHOICES 1 Fat

Calories 45 | Calories from Fat 40 | Total Fat 4.5 g | Saturated Fat 0.5 g | Trans Fat 0.0 g
Cholesterol 0 mg | Sodium 50 mg | Potassium 50 mg | Total Carbohydrate 2 g
Dietary Fiber 0 g | Sugars 1 g | Protein 1 g | Phosphorus 10 mg

indonesian sambal

 16 servings

 1 tablespoon

This sauce or sambal separates the men from the boys. Although removing the seeds from a pepper will make it less hot, this is a spicy, fiery condiment that is amazing when mixed with cucumbers, sliced cabbage, or carrots. It can be used as a base for kimchee (the spicy hot condiment used at almost every Korean meal) or mixed into cooked Chinese noodles or steamed rice. It will open your palate and certainly stimulate conversation around the dinner table.

1/2 cup chili peppers, halved and seeded (jalapeño, serrano, or Thai chili)

5 garlic cloves

1 tablespoon fresh ginger, minced

1 teaspoon Florida Crystals or sugar

1 teaspoon kosher or sea salt

1 tablespoon white vinegar

1 tablespoon lime juice

1 tablespoon cilantro, minced

1 Place all ingredients in a food processor fitted with the metal blade, or a blender and blend or process until smooth. Place in a jar with a tight-fitting lid and refrigerate up to two weeks. Makes about 1 cup.

EXCHANGES/CHOICES Free Food

Calories 5 | Calories from Fat 0 | Total Fat 0.0 g | Saturated Fat 0.0 g | Trans Fat 0.0 g
Cholesterol 0 mg | Sodium 120 mg | Potassium 20 mg | Total Carbohydrate 1 g
Dietary Fiber 0 g | Sugars 1 g | Protein 0 g | Phosphorus 0 mg

pure maple glaze

 32 servings

 1 tablespoon

Rich, earthy, and golden brown with caramel and nutty overtones, use this glaze to baste winter squash, or use sparingly as a salad dressing.

1 cup orange juice

1/4 cup pure maple syrup

Juice of 1 fresh lemon

1/2 teaspoon cinnamon

1 tablespoon tamari or soy sauce

2 tablespoons hazelnut or walnut oil

1 Combine all ingredients in a medium mixing bowl with a wire whisk. This all-purpose glaze will last for 2 weeks covered in your refrigerator.

 CHEF STEVE'S TIP:

Drizzle over shredded cabbage and carrots for an exotic slaw.
Brush apple slices and broil for a unique dinner garnish.
Use as a glaze to elevate acorn squash to star status.

EXCHANGES/CHOICES Free Food

Calories 20 | Calories from Fat 10 | Total Fat 1.0 g | Saturated Fat 0.1 g | Trans Fat 0.0 g
Cholesterol 0 mg | Sodium 30 mg | Potassium 25 mg | Total Carbohydrate 3 g
Dietary Fiber 0 g | Sugars 2 g | Protein 0 g | Phosphorus 0 mg

tuscan olive oil marinade

 6 servings

 1/6 recipe

This is a favorite "go to" recipe that has so many uses. It's a great dressing paired with all kinds of salad greens.

3 tablespoons good quality extra virgin olive oil

2 tablespoons balsamic vinegar

1 tablespoon lemon juice

2 cloves garlic, minced

2 teaspoons dried Italian herbs

1 teaspoon crushed fennel seeds

1/2 teaspoon dried red chili flakes

1/4 cup minced fresh herbs such as basil, oregano, tarragon, thyme, or rosemary

1/4 cup dry red wine, such as Chianti, Burgundy or Merlot (optional)

1 Combine all ingredients in a food processor or blend and purée until smooth.

CHEF STEVE'S TIP:

Try using it as a marinade for thick slices of firm tofu, on grilled vegetables, or simply on a raw vegetable salad. Drizzled on a sandwich or muffaletta (a favorite New Orleans sandwich typically made with ham, provolone cheese, salami, and a piquant olive salad), it's just incredibly delicious and versatile.

EXCHANGES/CHOICES 1 1/2 Fat

Calories 65 | Calories from Fat 65 | Total Fat 7.0 g | Saturated Fat 1.0 g | Trans Fat 0.0 g
Cholesterol 0 mg | Sodium 0 mg | Potassium 25 mg | Total Carbohydrate 1 g
Dietary Fiber 0 g | Sugars 0 g | Protein 0 g | Phosphorus 5 mg

creamy buttermilk **dill dressing**

 16 servings

 2 tablespoons

Wonderful on salads, grilled vegetables, or sandwiches.

1 cup plain fat-free Greek yogurt

1 cup low-fat buttermilk

1/4 cup fresh minced dill

1 tablespoon lemon juice

1 teaspoon sugar

1 teaspoon lemon pepper

1/2 teaspoon salt

1 Combine all ingredients in a food processor or blender and purée until smooth.

CHEF STEVE'S TIP:

Substitute fresh mint for dill and serve over fresh strawberries or blueberries.

EXCHANGES/CHOICES Free Food

Calories 15 | Calories from Fat 0 | Total Fat 0.0 g | Saturated Fat 0.1 g | Trans Fat 0.0 g
Cholesterol 0 mg | Sodium 120 mg | Potassium 60 mg | Total Carbohydrate 2 g
Dietary Fiber 0 g | Sugars 2 g | Protein 1 g | Phosphorus 40 mg

triple citrus **vinaigrette**

 6 servings

 1 ounce

This dressing can be used as a marinade for grilled vegetables, tofu, or tempeh. It's also perfect over mixed greens or sliced fresh fruit.

1/4 cup extra virgin olive oil

1 tablespoon Dijon-style mustard

1/2 cup orange juice

1/3 cup grapefruit juice

1/8 cup lemon or lime juice

1 tablespoon honey

2 teaspoons minced fresh gingerroot

1 tablespoon reduced-sodium soy sauce

2 teaspoons poppy seeds (optional)

1   Blend all ingredients in a food processor or blender until smooth. Dressing may be stored, covered, in refrigerator for up to 1 week.

EXCHANGES/CHOICES 1/2 Fruit | 2 Fat

Calories 110 | Calories from Fat 80 | Total Fat 9.0 g | Saturated Fat 1.3 g | Trans Fat 0.0 g
Cholesterol 0 mg | Sodium 155 mg | Potassium 80 mg | Total Carbohydrate 7 g
Dietary Fiber 0 g | Sugars 6 g | Protein 1 g | Phosphorus 10 mg

cooling raita sauce

 6 servings

 2 ounces

Raitas are quick yogurt-based sauces that are used as condiments for Indian-inspired entrées. This raita is excellent with spicy foods as the cucumber and mint cool your taste buds right down.

1 cup fat-free plain Greek yogurt

2 tablespoons fresh chopped mint leaves (substitute 1 tablespoon dried, only if necessary)

1/2 cup chopped, seeded, and peeled cucumber (English cucumbers work well)

1/4 cup minced red onion

1/2 teaspoon ground cumin

1/2 teaspoon salt, kosher, or sea salt

1/2 cup chopped, seeded tomato (optional)

1 Combine all ingredients well and refrigerate. Serve well chilled.

 CHEF STEVE'S TIP:

Serve this raita sauce with spicy dishes. It helps cool your palate down.

EXCHANGES/CHOICES Free food

Calories 20 | Calories from Fat 0 | Total Fat 0.0 g | Saturated Fat 0.1 g | Trans Fat 0.0 g
Cholesterol 0 mg | Sodium 190 mg | Potassium 115 mg | Total Carbohydrate 3 g
Dietary Fiber 0 g | Sugars 3 g | Protein 2 g | Phosphorus 70 mg

CHAPTER 7
Global Dips and Whirled Peas

I honestly remember when hummus was foreign to most people in the U.S. In the past decade, it has risen in popularity and now there are dozens of hummus flavors. Dips made with beans and other legumes are also in high demand. The truth is that every culture has its own signature dips and spreads made with healthy ingredients that make them delicious, protein-filled snacks. They are made without sweeteners, which makes beans and legume dips a "sweet" choice if you are watching and controlling your diet.

This is one of my favorite menu categories because the recipes keep well and can stay in the refrigerator a few days, ready for a quick power snack when you really need one. Creamy spreads are also forgiving and allow you to be creative and inspired. For example, **Broccomole** (page 120) resourcefully combines the best of two worlds in one dip. Guacamole and hummus marry perfectly to embrace crunchy broccoli florets in a culinary relationship that defies explanation but will live on in my repertoire. Because I am such a spicy food freak, I welcome the cooling, mouth-pleasing **Cucumber Yogurt Sauce** (page 124).

This collection of simple recipes makes eating and snacking more interesting and whimsical. These dips and spreads go well with fresh, seasonal, cut raw vegetables, which are great for your daily regimen.

broccomole

 10 servings

 1/2 cup

This is what you get when you take two of your most favorite foods, avocado and hummus, and marry them in the blender. Wonderful, creamy, and chunky at the same time. Forget the health implications here as we are combining broccoli, the king of cruciferous vegetables, with chickpeas and avocado. This di can be served as is, with chips, raw vegetables, and crackers or makes a killer flatbread pizza topped with a sprinkle of Jack and cheddar cheese.

2 cans (15 ounces each) chickpeas, rinsed

2 tablespoons tahini

2 cloves garlic, minced

2 ounces extra virgin olive oil

3 tablespoons fresh lemon juice

1 teaspoon cumin

2 teaspoons Tabasco

Sea salt, to taste

1/4 cup fat-free Greek yogurt

2 cups broccoli, rough chopped, blanched in steamer for 2 minutes (leave al dente)

1/2 ripe avocado

1 Combine all ingredients except broccoli and avocado in a food processor and blend, adding the broccoli last (leave broccoli a bit coarse).

2 Add 1/2 avocado and pulse for 1 second.

EXCHANGES/CHOICES 1 Carbohydrate | 1 High-Fat Meat

Calories 175 | Calories from Fat 90 | Total Fat 10.0 g | Saturated Fat 1.3 g
Trans Fat 0.0 g | Cholesterol 0 mg | Sodium 105 mg | Potassium 265 mg
Total Carbohydrate 17 g | Dietary Fiber 5 g | Sugars 3 g | Protein 6 g
Phosphorus 130 mg

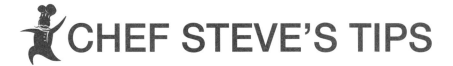

CHEF STEVE'S TIPS

hummus

- Hummus is rich in global culinary history and it takes many forms. (See recipe options listed on page 122.)

- In Greece, smashed chickpeas are served rustically, barely smashed with raw garlic and strong extra virgin olive oil poured over them. In many small tavernas, the chickpeas are served in a mortar and pestle and, as you sit at the table, you make the dish yourself.

- In parts of Italy, a form of hummus is made using white cannellini beans, lemon juice, caramelized garlic, and balsamic vinegar.

- Typical Middle Eastern hummus is always made with chickpeas, a sesame seed puree called tahini, lemon juice, garlic, and extra virgin olive oil. It is found on every street corner in Israel. And when people from Israel, Lebanon, or Turkey get together, it's always served.

- Commercially prepared hummus is pretty good. But it's really simple to make and so much better when you do it yourself. Once you make a "mother" batch of basic hummus, it can be flavored many ways.

- Hummus can be made in a food processor, blender or with an immersion blender.

basic hummus

 8 servings

 1/4 cup

Hummus, or finely mashed chickpeas, has to be one of the most perfect foods, especially if you are a vegetarian. Almost every nation makes some sort of bean purée. Hummus or any bean spread is an inexpensive protein source. And it is a wonderful summer dish that can be served over a salad, spread on flat bread, wrapped in tortillas, or scooped with raw vegetables. Hummus can be made in large batches and eaten all week.

2 cups canned chickpeas, rinsed well and drained

3 cloves garlic, chopped

3 tablespoons tahini

3 ice cubes

Juice of 1 lemon

1/2 teaspoon ground cumin

1/2 teaspoon hot sauce

Salt, to taste

1/4 cup extra virgin olive oil

1 Place chickpeas, garlic, tahini, ice cubes, lemon juice, cumin, hot sauce, and salt in a food processor fitted with the metal blade. Process until the mixture begins to become smooth. With the motor running, slowly add the olive oil through the feed tube until the mixture is creamy and smooth.

CHEF'S STEVE'S TIPS: HUMMUS VARIATIONS:

If you add three or four ice cubes when puréeing the chickpeas, they will emulsify the hummus faster, and you can use less oil.

Jalapeño and Scallion Hummus: Add 1 seeded, chopped jalapeño and 2 chopped scallions to the mixture before processing.

Kalamata Olive Hummus: Add 1/4 cup pitted kalamata olives to the mixture before processing. Or for a chunkier version, add the olives during the last 30 seconds of processing.

Roasted Red Pepper Hummus: Add 1/2 cup jarred roasted red pepper, drained very well, plus 1 teaspoon paprika to the mixture before processing.

EXCHANGES/CHOICES 1 Starch | 2 Fat

Calories 160 | Calories from Fat 100 | Total Fat 11.0 g | Saturated Fat 1.5 g
Trans Fat 0.0 g | Cholesterol 0 mg | Sodium 75 mg | Potassium 150 mg
Total Carbohydrate 13 g | Dietary Fiber 4 g | Sugars 2 g | Protein 4 g
Phosphorus 110 mg

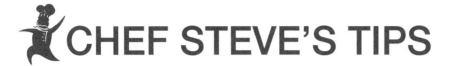# CHEF STEVE'S TIPS

yogurt

I use a lot of Greek yogurt in recipes as a healthier alternative to mayonnaise and sour cream. It can be used in dressings, sauces, to bind salads, and in desserts.

- Plain low-fat Greek yogurt is strained of excess liquid (which is mostly whey), so it is thick, dense, and creamy with an almost cream cheese–like texture.
- You can buy Greek yogurt in pints and larger containers, although it is incredibly easy to make. All you need is some paper towels or coffee filters and a colander.

To make Greek yogurt: Simply place colander in a mixing bowl and line it with a double layer of paper towels or a coffee filter. Dump a large container of plain, low-fat yogurt into the lined colander.

Lightly cover the bowl with plastic wrap so it doesn't absorb any additional flavors and refrigerate. The next day, the yogurt will be drained of liquid, which you can discard from the bowl. Return the drained yogurt to its original container or store it in another container.

cucumber yogurt sauce (tzatziki)

 6 servings

 1/6 recipe

In Greece, this sauce is a food group in itself. Use it to top grilled skewers of vegetables and chicken or a simple tossed salad or use as a dip for pita bread or freshly cut carrots and celery for a refreshing and delicious treat.

2 cucumbers, peeled, seeded, and grated

1 teaspoon kosher salt

2 tablespoons minced red onions

1 clove minced garlic

2 cups fat-free Greek-style yogurt

1 Place cucumbers in a colander in the sink and sprinkle with salt. Allow to drain 10 minutes. Rinse under cold running water to remove the salt. Press all the liquid out of the cucumbers.

2 Place cucumbers in a glass, stainless steel, or ceramic bowl with the remaining ingredients. Toss to combine.

 CHEF'S STEVE'S TIP:

Tzatziki is served in one form or another in almost every type of cuisine.

EXCHANGES/CHOICES 1/2 Fat-Free Milk

Calories 50 | Calories from Fat 0 | Total Fat 0.0 g | Saturated Fat 0.0 g | Trans Fat 0.0 g | Cholesterol 0 mg | Sodium 190 mg | Potassium 160 mg | Total Carbohydrate 5 g | Dietary Fiber 0 g | Sugars 4 g | Protein 8 g | Phosphorus 115 mg

double apple **pomegranate salsa**

 6 servings

 1/6 recipe

This salsa is juicy, tart, and a perfect accompaniment for grilled vegetables, tofu, or simply served on toasted French bread with a schmear of goat cheese for an appetizer.

2 apples, unpeeled, such as Granny Smith, Gala, Fuji, or Pink Lady, diced into 1/2-inch cubes

Juice of 1 lemon

1 tablespoon honey or agave syrup

1 tablespoon light brown sugar

1 small jalapeño pepper, seeded and minced

1 cup fresh pomegranate seeds

1/4 cup dried apples, chopped

1/4 cup unsweetened pomegranate juice

1. Combine all ingredients in a medium mixing bowl and allow the flavors to marry for at least a half hour or overnight in the refrigerator.

CHEF'S STEVE'S TIP:

You can now buy frozen pomegranate seeds, which make a good substitute and save time.

EXCHANGES/CHOICES 1 1/2 Fruit

Calories 95 | Calories from Fat 0 | Total Fat 0.0 g | Saturated Fat 0.1 g | Trans Fat 0.0 g
Cholesterol 0 mg | Sodium 10 mg | Potassium 210 mg | Total Carbohydrate 24 g
Dietary Fiber 3 g | Sugars 19 g | Protein 1 g | Phosphorus 25 mg

watermelon, feta, and mint salsa

 6 servings

 1/6 recipe

Scoop up this summery spicy salsa as a dip with tortilla or pita chips. Or, better yet, eat it with a spoon!

2 cups watermelon, seeded and diced into 1/2-inch cubes

1/2 cup low-fat feta cheese

1/2 cup yellow pepper, chopped

1/4 cup red onion, minced

1 each jalapeño or serrano chili, seeded and minced

1/4 cup mint leaves, chopped

1/4 cup parsley, chopped

1 tablespoon fresh squeezed lemon juice

1 Combine all ingredients well in a medium mixing bowl. Allow flavors to combine for at least 15 minutes.

 CHEF STEVE'S TIP:

Try a Latin variation. Substitute:
cilantro for mint
lime juice for lemon
queso blanco for feta cheese

EXCHANGES/CHOICES 1/2 Carbohydrate

Calories 30 | Calories from Fat 0 | Total Fat 0.0 g | Saturated Fat 0.0 g | Trans Fat 0.0 g
Cholesterol 0 mg | Sodium 0 mg | Potassium 150 mg | Total Carbohydrate 7 g
Dietary Fiber 1 g | Sugars 4 g | Protein 1 g | Phosphorus 15 mg

caesar **salsa**

 10 servings

 2 ounces

Like a bite-size Caesar salad, this is an incredible sandwich topper with grilled tempeh or tofu.

4 cups romaine, sliced very thin julienne

2 cloves garlic, minced

1/8 cup freshly shredded Parmesan or Romano cheese

2 teaspoons light mayonnaise

1 teaspoon Dijon mustard

1 Mix all ingredients together well. Must be served immediately.

EXCHANGES/CHOICES Free Food

Calories 10 | Calories from Fat 5 | Total Fat 0.5 g | Saturated Fat 0.2 g | Trans Fat 0.0 g
Cholesterol 0 mg | Sodium 35 mg | Potassium 50 mg | Total Carbohydrate 1 g
Dietary Fiber 0 g | Sugars 0 g | Protein 1 g | Phosphorus 15 mg

punjabi-style salsa

 10 servings

 2 ounces

Fiery, sweet, and pungent, this salsa will electrify your taste buds and add vibrant color to your dinner plates. You may use jalapeño, Anaheim, or Scotch bonnet chilis, depending on your heat tolerance.

2 cups chopped tomato

1 cup chopped mango, papaya, or peach

1 teaspoon minced gingerroot

1 tablespoon fresh minced chilies

2 tablespoons lime juice

2 tablespoons fresh minced cilantro

1 Mix all ingredients well and store refrigerated.

 CHEF STEVE'S TIP:

Toss with cooked, whole-grain pasta or cooked brown rice.

EXCHANGES/CHOICES Free Food

Calories 20 | Calories from Fat 0 | Total Fat 0.0 g | Saturated Fat 0.0 g | Trans Fat 0.0 g
Cholesterol 0 mg | Sodium 0 mg | Potassium 120 mg | Total Carbohydrate 5 g
Dietary Fiber 1 g | Sugars 3 g | Protein 0 g | Phosphorus 10 mg

picnic salsa

 10 servings

 2 ounces

This salsa screams summer, but is welcome year round.

1 cup chopped watermelon

1/2 cup chopped cantaloupe

1/2 cup chopped, peeled cucumbers

1 cup chopped tomatoes

1/2 cup chopped green peppers

1 tablespoon jalapeño or serrano chilies, seeded and minced

2 tablespoons minced parsley or cilantro

2 tablespoons lemon juice

1 Combine all ingredients well and store in a covered bowl in the refrigerator.

EXCHANGES/CHOICES Free Food

Calories 15 | Calories from Fat 0 | Total Fat 0.0 g | Saturated Fat 0.0 g | Trans Fat 0.0 g
Cholesterol 0 mg | Sodium 0 mg | Potassium 115 mg | Total Carbohydrate 3 g
Dietary Fiber 1 g | Sugars 2 g | Protein 0 g | Phosphorus 10 mg

kiwi-corn **salsa**

 10 servings

 2 ounces

The combination of corn and kiwi is both colorful and complementary. Try it in a burrito or quesdilla.

4 ripe kiwis, peeled and cut into 1/4-inch dice

1 small ripe papaya or 2 ripe peaches, cut into 1/4-inch dice

1 ripe tomato, cut into 1/4-inch dice

1 cup corn kernels, frozen, or 2 ears fresh, lightly steamed and cut from the cob

2 tablespoons corn oil

2 tablespoons lime juice

2 tablespoons cilantro, minced

1 Combine all ingredients well and store in a covered container in the refrigerator.

EXCHANGES/CHOICES 1/2 Fruit | 1/2 Fat

Calories 65 | Calories from Fat 25 | Total Fat 3.0 g | Saturated Fa 0.4 g | Trans Fat 0.0 g
Cholesterol 0 mg | Sodium 0 mg | Potassium 200 mg | Total Carbohydrate 9 g
Dietary Fiber 2 g | Sugars 4 g | Protein 1 g | Phosphorus 25 mg

salsa **minestrone**

 10 servings

 3 ounces

Wonderful on any Mediterranean dish, the colors and textures in this salsa make any dish worthy of company.

1 ripe tomato, chopped

1/3 cup minced red onion

1 cup zucchini, diced in 1/4-inch dice

1 cup chopped green cabbage

1/2 cup chopped red pepper

6 chopped black kalamata olives

2 tablespoons extra virgin olive oil

1/8 cup red wine vinegar

1/2 cup chopped basil

1/2 cup minced parsley

1 teaspoon fennel seeds, crushed

1 teaspoon oregano dried

1/2 teaspoon kosher or sea salt

1 Combine all ingredients well and store covered in refrigerator.

 CHEF STEVE'S TIP:

Serve as a dip with tortilla chips, or fold into cooked whole-wheat pasta.

EXCHANGES/CHOICES 1 Vegetable | 1/2 Fat

Calories 45 | Calories from Fat 30 | Total Fat 3.5 g | Saturated Fat 0.4 g | Trans Fat 0.0 g
Cholesterol 0 mg | Sodium 120 mg | Potassium 140 mg | Total Carbohydrate 3 g
Dietary Fiber 1 g | Sugars 2 g | Protein 1 g | Phosphorus 20 mg

broccoli black bean hummus

 12 servings

 2 ounces

This hummus has a twist—it's crunchy and has added antioxidants. Tahini or sesame paste can be found in all natural food stores and Asian food markets. Most supermarkets now carry it as well. If desired, add 1 tablespoon of minced cilantro.

3 cups broccoli florets

1 (16-ounce) can chickpeas, well rinsed and drained

1 cup plain, fat-free yogurt

1/4 cup tahini (sesame seed paste)

2 cloves garlic, minced

3 each scallions, minced

2 teaspoons Tabasco sauce

1/2 teaspoon cumin, ground

1 teaspoon kosher salt

Juice of 1 lemon or lime

1 (16-ounce) can black beans, well rinsed and drained

1 Trim broccoli into small florets, reserving stems for another use. Steam florets over boiling water for 3–4 minutes until still crisp, rinse under cold water and reserve, or microwave on high in about 1/2 inch water for 2 minutes and rinse under cold water. Set aside.

2 Place 1 cup of the cooked broccoli in a food processor fitted with the standard blade. The additional 2 cups will be added later. Add all ingredients except the black beans in the food processor and process until fairly smooth but still showing some pieces. Add the remaining broccoli florets, saving a few for garnish, and the black beans. Process using the pulse button, once or twice only until incorporated.

EXCHANGES/CHOICES 1 Starch | 1/2 Fat

Calories 110 | Calories from Fat 30 | Total Fat 3.5 g | Saturated Fat 0.5 g | Trans Fat 0.0 g | Cholesterol 0 mg | Sodium 255 mg | Potassium 285 mg | Total Carbohydrate 15 g | Dietary Fiber 5 g | Sugars 4 g | Protein 6 g | Phosphorus 150 mg

skordalia (potato dip)

 12 servings

 1/4 cup

This dip is traditionally made by hand. You can make it that way, but I prefer to use a food processor. It's wonderful on sandwiches, as a dip, or served with warm flatbread.

5 peeled Idaho baking potatoes

Water for cooking potatoes

5 cloves garlic, minced

1 teaspoon kosher salt

1/2 cup good-quality Greek or Italian extra virgin olive oil

1/4 cup fresh lemon juice

2 tablespoons water

1 Place potatoes in a large pot of water and bring to a boil. Cook 30 minutes until tender, drain, and set aside to cool 15 minutes.

2 Holding the potatoes with a kitchen towel, peel, break up, and place in a food processor fitted with the metal blade. Add garlic and salt. Use on/off pulses until the mixture is just combined. Be careful not to over-process as the potatoes will get glutinous and tough. Add the olive oil, lemon juice, and water and again use on/off pulses until just combined and smooth.

EXCHANGES/CHOICES 1 Starch | 1 1/2 Fat

Calories 135 | Calories from Fat 80 | Total Fat 9.0 g | Saturated Fat 1.3 g | Trans Fat 0.0 g
Cholesterol 0 mg | Sodium 165 mg | Potassium 245 mg | Total Carbohydrate 13 g
Dietary Fiber 1 g | Sugars 1g | Protein 1 g | Phosphorus 30 mg

CHAPTER 8
Desserts

Of all the recipe challenges when managing diabetes, I think desserts take the most planning. Personally, I would rather rely on the natural sweetness of fruits, vegetables, and other ingredients before I use other forms of sweeteners.

With that said, you'll find the desserts in this section simple to prepare, light, and appropriate for all seasons, even as the produce selection changes. In order to offer great desserts that leave no crave factor, I thoughtfully added ingredients that satisfy and tingle the taste buds, such as fresh ginger root, cinnamon, cardamom, mint, and balsamic vinegar. Many of the recipes are dual purpose as they can clearly be served as a more traditional dessert course, while others like the **Balsamic Strawberries** (page 136) and the **Free-Form Tropical Fruit Ambrosia Salad** (page 141) double as an appetizer to begin your meal. For those of you who love to man the grill, don't stop at grilling pineapple as presented in the **Spice Market Grill Pan Pineapple Steaks** (page 142). Feel free to go outside and fire up the grill using any firm seasonal fruit. When firm fruit is grilled outside over gas or wood, its flavor intensifies and it takes on a delicate, smoky flavor that makes a wonderful dessert.

balsamic **strawberries**

 4 servings

 3/4 cup

These tart berries, with a bit of freshly ground black pepper, are incredible over vanilla bean ice cream. Although at first glance the combination sounds unusual, it's sure to become a dinner table tradition.

1 pint fresh strawberries, rinsed, hulled, and halved

1 teaspoon Splenda

1 tablespoon good-quality balsamic vinegar

Freshly ground black pepper, to taste

4 (1/2-cup) scoops sugar-free vanilla bean ice cream

1 Combine the berries, Splenda, vinegar, and pepper in a mixing bowl and chill 30 minutes. Serve over ice cream.

EXCHANGES/CHOICES 1 1/2 Carbohydrate | 1/2 Fat

Calories 130 | Calories from Fat 30 | Total Fat 3.5 g | Saturated Fat 2.0 g | Trans Fat 0.0 g | Cholesterol 10 mg | Sodium 30 mg | Potassium 270 mg | Total Carbohydrate 22 g | Dietary Fiber 4 g | Sugars 8 g | Protein 4 g | Phosphorus 75 mg

berry, chocolate, **and vanilla soy strata**

 6 servings

 1 cup

This desset has layers and layers of guilt-free flavor, creamy texture, and juicy berries. Make this a day ahead to let the flavors melt into one another. Use a clear straight-sided glass bowl for the best visual presentation. Feel free to make a tropical version using layers of papaya, mango, pineapple, and banana. Sprinkle with a bit of coconut as well.

1 cup unsweetened chocolate soy or almond milk

1 cup unsweetened vanilla soy or almond milk

2 tablespoons Splenda, divided in half

4 tablespoons of cornstarch divided in half, each mixed with a tablespoon of cold soy or almond milk

1 pint raspberries

1 pint blackberries

1 pint strawberries, hulled and sliced

Cocoa powder (for garnish)

1 Heat the soy milk flavors in separate pots over low heat. Add 1 tablespoon of Splenda and 2 tablespoons of cornstarch mixed with cold soy milk to each pot of simmering soy milk and heat until the milk thickens. Remove from the heat and cool.

2 In a large glass bowl, layer the chocolate and vanilla soy milk with the berries forming layers. End up with a layer of berries on top and sprinkle with cocoa powder.

EXCHANGES/CHOICES 1 Carbohydrate | 1/2 Fat

Calories 105 | Calories from Fat 15 | Total Fat 1.5 g | Saturated Fat 0.2 g | Trans Fat 0.0 g
Cholesterol 0 mg | Sodium 45 mg | Potassium 315 mg | Total Carbohydrate 21 g
Dietary Fiber 8 g | Sugars 8 g | Protein 4 g | Phosphorus 120 mg

pear and stilton cobbler **with pecans**

 12 servings

 1/12 cobbler

Stilton is an imported English member of the blue cheese family. It is strong in flavor and goes quite well with sweet pears. Use domestic blue cheese or cheddar, if you prefer. Use pears that are ripe but not soft, preferably Anjou or green pears.

BOTTOM FRUIT LAYER

8 Anjou pears, peeled, cored, and cut into 1-inch cubes

Juice of 1 lemon (zest first and reserve for batter)

1 tablespoon cornstarch

1/4 cup crumbled Stilton or blue cheese

1 teaspoon almond extract

Pinch salt

COBBLER BATTER

7 tablespoons light butter canola oil blend or light butter (such as Land O' Lakes), softened

1/4 cup egg substitute

1/4 cup Splenda Brown Sugar Blend

1 1/4 cups whole-wheat flour

1/2 cup old-fashioned rolled oats

2 teaspoons baking soda

1/2 teaspoon salt

1/2 cup low-fat buttermilk

1 teaspoon lemon peel or zest

1/4 cup pecan pieces

TO MAKE FRUIT LAYER

1 Preheat oven to 350°F. In a large bowl, combine pears, lemon juice, cornstarch, Stilton cheese, almond extract, and salt. Place in a 2-quart ovenproof nonreactive dish.

TO MAKE BATTER

2 In a medium bowl, using an electric hand mixer or whisk, beat together butter and brown sugar until smooth. Add egg and beat to combine well.

3 In another bowl, combine flour, oats, baking soda, and salt. Add half the flour mixture to butter mixture and beat to combine. Mix in half the buttermilk and mix to combine. Add remaining flour mixture and combine. Mix in remaining buttermilk, lemon zest, and pecans.

4 Spread batter on top of fruit layer in pan and bake 45 minutes.

EXCHANGES/CHOICES 2 Carbohydrate | 1 Fat

Calories 205 | Calories from Fat 55 | Total Fat 6.0 g | Saturated Fat 2.0 g | Trans Fat 0.0 g
Cholesterol 5 mg | Sodium 435 mg | Potassium 255 mg | Total Carbohydrate 35 g
Dietary Fiber 6 g | Sugars 14 g | Protein 4 g | Phosphorus 100 mg

butternut squash and apple bread

 12 servings

 1 slice

Moist and tender, this breakfast bread is incredible spread with cream cheese or preserves. You can make muffins out of the mix by dividing the batter into a muffin tin, if you wish.

1 cup all-purpose flour

1/2 cup Splenda brown sugar blend

1 teaspoon cinnamon

1 teaspoon allspice

1 teaspoon salt

2 teaspoons baking powder

1/3 cup chopped walnuts or pecans

1/3 cup sun-dried cranberries

1 (1-pound) package frozen butternut squash, thawed

2 eggs, lightly beaten

1 cup unsweetened applesauce

1/3 cup apple juice or skim milk

1. Preheat oven to 350°F. Lightly grease a 9 × 5 × 3-inch loaf pan.

2. Combine flour, sugar, spices, baking powder, nuts, cranberries, and squash in a large mixing bowl.

3. Combine eggs, applesauce, and apple juice or milk in another bowl.

4. Make a well in the center of the dry ingredients and pour in wet ingredients. Fold in until just combined.

5. Pour into prepared pan and bake in the center of the oven 1 hour until baked through or until a toothpick inserted into the center comes out clean. If baked as muffins, cooking time will be approximately 30 minutes.

EXCHANGES/CHOICES 2 Carbohydrate

Calories 140 | Calories from Fat 25 | Total Fat 3.0 g | Saturated Fat 0.5 g | Trans Fat 0.0 g
Cholesterol 30 mg | Sodium 270 mg | Potassium 125 mg | Total Carbohydrate 26
Dietary Fiber 2 g | Sugars 9 g | Protein 3 g | Phosphorus 125 mg

apple pecan brown betty

 6 servings

 1/6 recipe

There is nothing better than being the first person to crack open the rolled oat crust, exposing the aromatic apples and cranberries underneath.

6 apples, peeled, and sliced in 1/4-inch slices (Fuji, Gala, or Red Delicious variety)

1 teaspoon ground cinnamon, divided use

1/2 teaspoon nutmeg

1 teaspoon almond extract

2 tablespoons Splenda and brown sugar mix, divided use

6 ounces unsweetened cranberry juice

2 tablespoons dried cranberries

1 teaspoon balsamic vinegar

2 slices whole-grain bread

1/4 cup quick-cooking oats

1 tablespoon butter blend (such as Land O' Lakes or Brummel & Brown)

2 tablespoons chopped pecans or walnuts

1 Preheat oven to 350°F.

2 In a medium saucepot, combine apples, 1/2 teaspoon of the cinnamon, nutmeg, almond extract, 1 tablespoon of the Splenda Brown Sugar Blend, cranberry juice, cranberries, and balsamic vinegar over medium-high heat. Cook approximately 10 minutes until softened but not mushy.

3 Remove from heat and transfer to a 9-inch glass or Pyrex pie plate.

4 Process whole-grain bread in food processor until coarse crumbs are made. Use pulse function to make sure they are not too fine.

5 Combine breadcrumbs, oats, butter blend, nuts, remaining Splenda blend, and remaining cinnamon in a small bowl.

6 Sprinkle crumb mixture over apples and bake uncovered for 20–25 minutes until lightly browned.

EXCHANGES/CHOICES 2 Carbohydrate | 1 Fat

Calories 175 | Calories from Fat 40 | Total Fat 4.5 g | Saturated Fat 1.0 g | Trans Fat 0.0 g
Cholesterol 5 mg | Sodium 60 mg | Potassium 190 mg | Total Carbohydrate 34 g
Dietary Fiber 3 g | Sugars 21 g | Protein 2 g | Phosphorus 60 mg

free-form tropical fruit **ambrosia salad**

 4 servings

 1/4 recipe

This isn't like the ambrosia I grew up with on the school cafeteria line; this one is light, refreshing, and appropriate to start or finish any meal.

1 large pink grapefruit, peel removed and cut into large cubes

2 navel oranges, peel removed and cut into large cubes

1 cup papaya, peeled and cut into large cubes

1 kiwi, peeled and cut into large cubes

8 strawberries, stem removed and quartered

1 2/3 tablespoons dried and flaked unsweetened coconut

1 tablespoon honey or agave

1 Combine all ingredients in a medium mixing bowl and toss. Marinate for 20 minutes before serving for best flavor.

EXCHANGES/CHOICES 1 1/2 Fruit | 1/2 Fat

Calories 110 | Calories from Fat 20 | Total Fat 2.0 g | Saturated Fat 1.4 g | Trans Fat 0.0 g
Cholesterol 0 mg | Sodium 0 mg | Potassium 380 mg | Total Carbohydrate 24 g
Dietary Fiber 4 g | Sugars 18 g | Protein 2 g | Phosphorus 30 mg

spice market grill pan pineapple steaks

 4 servings

 1/4 recipe

Serve these pineapple "steaks" warm over sugar-free vanilla ice cream or coconut sorbet for a memorable sweet ending.

1 medium pineapple, cored and sliced 1/2-inch thick

Juice of 1 lime

2 teaspoons honey

1 teaspoon vanilla

1/4 teaspoon cardamom, ground

1/8 teaspoon clove, ground

1/2 teaspoon cinnamon, ground

Spray butter or butter-flavored oil for grill pan

1 Marinate pineapple slices with all ingredients in a covered pan in the refrigerator for up to 8 hours, prior to preparing.

2 Heat a grill pan over medium-high heat and then spray with butter-flavored spray or butter spray. Grill pineapple slices for 1–2 minutes, then turn over and repeat process until grill marked and heated through.

EXCHANGES/CHOICES 1 Fruit

Calories 75 | Calories from Fat 0 | Total Fat 0.0 g | Saturated Fat 0.0 g | Trans Fat 0.0 g
Cholesterol 0 mg | Sodium 0 mg | Potassium 140 mg | Total Carbohydrate 19 g
Dietary Fiber 2 g | Sugars 15 g | Protein 1 g | Phosphorus 10 mg

minted fruit salsa **with cinnamon chips**

 4 servings

 1/4 recipe

What a perfect couple these two recipes make! The crispy cinnamon chips can also be used with any of your other favorite dips.

1/2 cup pineapple, diced in cubes

1 kiwi, diced in cubes

1/2 cup strawberries, diced

1/2 cup melon (either cantaloupe or honeydew)

1 navel orange, peeled and diced

1/4 cup fresh raspberries

2 teaspoons lime juice

1 tablespoon sugar-free orange marmalade

1 tablespoon fresh mint leaves, minced

1 Combine all ingredients well in a mixing bowl and marinate for 10 minutes before serving. Scoop salsa with Cinnamon Baked Tortilla Chips below.

EXCHANGES/CHOICES 1 Fruit

Calories 60 | Calories from Fat 0 | Total Fat 0.0 g | Saturated Fat 0.0 g | Trans Fat 0.0 g
Cholesterol 0 mg | Sodium 5 mg | Potassium 250 mg | Total Carbohydrate 16 g
Dietary Fiber 3 g | Sugars 11g | Protein 1 g | Phosphorus 25 mg

CINNAMON BAKED TORTILLA CHIPS

2 (10-inch) whole-wheat flour tortillas, cut into 2-inch-wide strips

vegetable oil for spraying

1 tablespoon Florida Crystals or light brown sugar

1/2 teaspoon cinnamon

1 Heat oven to 350°F. Place tortilla strips on a baking pan.

2 Spray with oil and sprinkle with sugar and cinnamon.

3 Bake for 12 minutes until golden brown.

EXCHANGES/CHOICES 1 1/2 Starch

Calories 110 | Calories from Fat 5 | Total Fat 0.5 g
Saturated Fat 0.1 g | Trans Fat 0.0 g | Cholesterol 0 mg
Sodium 170 mg | Potassium 90 mg | Total Carbohydrate 23 g
Dietary Fiber 3 g | Sugars 3 g | Protein 3 g | Phosphorus 75 mg

gingered summer fruit sauce

 6 servings

 1/6 recipe

Use any seasonal fruit and this recipe becomes the perfect dessert sauce year round. The spicy ginger perks up this sauce and makes it memorable.

2 ounces honey

4 ounces apple juice

1 teaspoon ginger, grated

1 cinnamon stick

2 pounds peaches, plums, or nectarines, pitted and sliced into 1/2-inch-thick wedges

2 teaspoons cornstarch dissolved in water or apple juice

Juice of 1/2 lemon

1 In a saucepan over moderate heat, bring honey, apple juice, ginger, and cinnamon stick to a boil.

2 Add sliced fruit and simmer for approximately 3–5 minutes until fruit is softened but still retains its character. Add cornstarch dissolved in liquid and lemon juice. Stir until thickened, about 2 minutes.

3 Serve this fruit sauce warm over frozen yogurt, angel food cake, or lemon sorbet. If desired, a combination of summer fruits may be used.

EXCHANGES/CHOICES 1 Fruit | 1/2 Carbohydrate

Calories 100 | Calories from Fat 0 | Total Fat 0.0 g | Saturated Fat 0.0 g | Trans Fat 0.0 g
Cholesterol 0 mg | Sodium 0 mg | Potassium 65 mg | Total Carbohydrate 25 g
Dietary Fiber 2 g | Sugars 22 g | Protein 1 g | Phosphorus 25 mg

CHAPTER 9
Menu Suggestions

BUILDING A MEAL 101

Assembling the components of a meal used to be the equivalent of planning the seating arrangements for a wedding. One had to be overly careful that all the guests seated together got along and could be civil for a few hours. There were so many concerns over the event going terribly wrong if a miscalculation was made. When it comes to meal planning, that has changed. In fact, all the dishes in this book are totally vegetarian, plus there is much thought surrounding the use of eclectic, bold, and global flavors. That's not to say that a certain food and common sense needs to be considered when combining recipes to make a meal. Go ahead and be creative with your menu pairings. Think of the following suggestions as flavor groupings, incorporating recipes that enhance each other. There are various ethnic groupings that make sense as well as combining dishes by holiday, textural partners, and even colors.

On a hot, sunny day, Caribbean dishes make sense, while on a chilly winter weekend, a hearty stew, a crunchy salad with creamy buttermilk dressing, and a warm loaf of bread fits the bill. Flavor first is my motto and the rest will fall into place! Here are a few of my personal favorite flavor profiles and menus that you'll want to test-drive.

WINTER CRAVINGS:

- Creamy White Bean Soup with Basil and Olive Oil (page 21)
- Endive Salad with Stilton, Pear, and Walnuts (page 28)
- Acorn Squash Stuffed with Apple, Almond, Cranberry Basmati Pilaf (page 56)

GO GREEK:

- Greek Egg and Lemon Soup (page 14)
- Spinach, Rosemary, and Garlic Cakes (page 49)
- Athenian-Style Roast Zucchinni (page 86)

TUSCAN TOSS UP:

- Watercress, Golden Beets, and Fennel Salad with Parmesan-Peppercorn Dressing (page 35)
- Creamy Cavatappi ~ Tuscan Mac n' Cheese (page 76)
- Balsamic Strawberries (page 136)

BOUNTY WITHOUT BORDER:

- Five Alarm Garden Chili (page 23)
- Terra Cotta Cobb Salad (page 30)
- Grilled Tofu or Tempeh with Avocado Chili Salsa (page 81)

ASIAN FLING:

- Singapore Cucumber Salad (page 34)
- Pan Seared Spicy Asparagus with Shiitake Mushrooms (page 60)
- Sticky Brown Rice Cakes (page 52)

MADRAS MENU:

- Basil Ginger Cashew Pilaf (page 57)
- Smoky Chickpeas with Spinach, Eggplant, Tomato, and Manchego Cheese (page 62)
- Punjabi-Style Salsa (page 128)

CARIBEAN BREEZE:

- Grapefruit and Avocado Salad with Honey Mustard Citrus Dressing (page 41)
- Trinidadian Curry Vegetables (page 65)
- Spice Market Grill Pan Pineapple Steaks (page 142)

alphabetical index

A

acorn squash stuffed with apple-almond-cranberry basmati pilaf, 56
apple pecan brown betty, 140
Athenian-style roast zucchini, 86
autumn skillet paella, 74
avocado chili salsa, 82

B

bagna cauda, 108
balsamic strawberries, 136
barely cooked tomatoes with basil and whole-grain pasta, 75
barley and corn strata salad in mason jars, 37
basic hummus, 122
basil ginger cashew pilaf, 57
berry, chocolate, and vanilla soy strata, 137
black bean patties with cilantro and lime, 45
broccoli black bean hummus, 132
broccomole, 120
butternut squash and apple bread, 139

C

Caesar salsa, 127
campfire corn and black bean salad, 38
cauliflower potato cheddar mash, 87
Chef Steve's diablo dipping sauce, 112
chef's surprise package, 72
cherry almond couscous, 93
chicpea and hominy stew, 22
chicpea pancakes with cilantro, 92
chimichurri cilantro sauce, 111
Claire's retro stuffed peppers, 58
coco rice with green onion, 100
cooling raita sauce, 118
couscous and feta cakes, 46
cowboy style "meatloaf", 47
creamy buttermilk dill dressing, 116
creamy cavatappi ~ Tuscan mac n' cheese, 76
creamy white bean soup with basil and olive oil, 21
crunchy cajun cabbage slaw, 39
cucumber, pineapple, and papaya salsa, 110
cucumber yogurt sauce (tzatziki), 124

D

double apple pomegranate salsa, 125

E

eggplant risotto cakes, 48
emerald sesame kale, 104
endive salad with stilton, pear, and walnuts, 28
energizing minestrone, 10
enlightened tub of noodles, 59

F

feelin' your oats burgers, 44
festive vegetable gateau, 88
fire-roasted tomato florentine, 101
five alarm garden chili, 23
flash in the pan veggies, 103
free-form tropical fruit ambrosia salad, 141

G

garden party roast vegetables with pasta, 77
garlic spinach, 89
ginger soy drizzle, 109
gingered summer fruit sauce, 144
grapefruit and avocado salad with honey mustard citrus dressing, 41
Greek egg and lemon soup, 14
green velvet chilled avocado soup, 20
grilled asparagus with sun-dried tomatoes and parmesan, 99
grilled tofu (or tempeh) with avocado chili salsa, 81

H

herb-crusted tofu with fresh herb salsa verde, 78
herbed spaetzel, 18
herbed spaetzel and lentil soup, 17
holiday yucca stew with black beans, cilantro, and lime, 12

I

Indonesian sambal, 113

K

kiwi-corn salsa, 130

subject index

grilling, 135
guacamole, 119

H
harissa, 6
herb-crusted tofu with fresh herb salsa verde, 78
herbed spaetzel, 18
herbed spaetzel and lentil soup, 17
herbs, 17–18, 115
hoisin sauce, 6
holiday yucca stew with black beans, cilantro, and lime, 12
hominy, 22, 80
honey, 41, 144
hummus, 119, 121

I
ice cream, 136
Indonesian sambal, 113
Italian food, 121, 146

J
jalapeño peppers, 23, 65, 111, 125, 129
Jerusalem artichoke, 35

K
kalamata olives, 33
kale, 22, 39, 104–105
kiwi, 130, 141, 143
kiwi-corn salsa, 130

L
lacto-ovo vegetarian, 4
latke, 94
legumes, 5
lemon caper sauce, 73
lemon/lemon juice, 14, 31, 71, 73, 108, 114, 117
lentil dal, 24
lentils, 5, 17, 24
lime/lime juice, 12, 30, 45, 83, 142
loaded twice-baked potatoes, 67
lots of vegetable soup, 19
luscious avocado-strawberry salad with toasted pine nuts, 29

M
Madras food, 146
maple syrup, 114

marcona almonds, 16
marinade, 107, 115
marinara sauce, 58, 84
mason jars, 37
meal planning, 55, 145–146
menu suggestions, 145–146
Middle Eastern food, 121
mint leaves, 33, 118, 126
minted chickpeas and feta with kalamata olives, 33
minted fruit salsa with cinnamon chips, 143
Mirin (rice wine), 34
miso-noodle soup, 25
mole marinara sauce, 84
mushrooms, 53, 60, 79
mustard, 6

N
New Year's lucky round risotto, 90
nuts. See *under specific type*

O
oats, 44, 47, 140
oils, 6
olive oil, 6, 21, 115
orange/orange juice, 41, 114, 117, 141, 143
oregano, 108

P
pan-roasted harvest root vegetables, 102
pan-seared shredded brussels sprouts and apples, 95
pan-seared tofu with garlic and lime & watercress, 83
pancake, 92
pan-seared spicy asparagus with shiitake mushrooms, 60
pantry, 5
papaya, 110, 128, 130, 141
parmesan, 99
parsley leaves, 111
parsnip, 19, 102
pasta, 5
    cavatappi, 76
    cavatelli, 26
    energizing minestrone, 10
    enlightened tub of noodles, 59
    miso-noodle soup, 25
    pasta con fagioli, 26
    pasta pomodoro, 61
    ravioli, 68

T

tahini, 122
tamari, 6
tempeh, 7, 69, 73, 81
terra cotta cobb salad, 30
textured vegetable protein, 69
the mother rice pilaf, 91
tofu, 7, 15, 31, 69–70, 72, 78, 81, 83
tofu nicoise salad, 31
tomatoes, 24, 61–62, 75, 82, 86, 101, 128, 131
tortilla chips, 15, 143
tortilla soup with black beans and chilies, 15
Trinidadian curry vegetables, 65
triple citrus vinaigrette, 117
turnip, 102
Tuscan olive oil marinade, 115
twice cooked sweet potato croquettes, 50, 54

U

udon noodle pancakes with shiitake mushrooms, 53

V

vegan, 4
vegetable. *See also under specific type*
    autumn skillet paella, 74
    chef's surprise package, 72
    energizing minestrone, 10
    enlightened tub of noodles, 59
    festive vegetable gateau, 88
    five-alarm garden chili, 23
    flash in the pan veggies, 103
    garden party roast vegetables with pasta, 77

    lots of vegetable soup, 19
    miso-noodle soup, 25
    pan roasted harvest root vegetables, 102
    Steve's super bowl of garden chili, 66
    Trinidadian curry vegetables, 65
vegetarian classifications, 4
vegetarian pantry, 5
vinegars, 6

W

walnut, 28, 44, 50, 54
water chestnuts, 53
watercress, 35, 83
watercress, golden beets and fennel salad with parmesan-peppercorn dressing, 35
watermelon, 126, 129
watermelon, feta, and mint salsa, 126
wheat gluten, 7
white gazpacho with marcona almonds and grapes, 16

Y

yogurt, 16, 67, 123
yogurt, Greek, 20, 116, 118, 123–124
yucca, 12

Z

zucchini, 63–64, 86, 88, 131
zucchini, sweet pepper, and soy sausage pilaf, 63
zucchini with rigatoni, pine nuts, and sun-dried tomatoes, 64